MICROCOSM PUBLISHING

Microcosm Publishing is Portland's most diversified publishing house and distributor with a focus on the colorful, authentic, and empowering. Our books and zines have put your power in your hands since 1996, equipping readers to make positive changes in their lives and in the world around them. Microcosm emphasizes skill-building, showing hidden histories, and fostering creativity through challenging conventional publishing wisdom with books and bookettes about DIY skills, food, bicycling, gender, self-care, and social justice. What was once a distro and record label was started by Joe Biel in his bedroom and has become among the oldest independent publishing houses in Portland, OR. We are a politically moderate, centrist publisher in a world that has inched to the right for the past 80 years.

Contents

Acknowledgements

To my sprogs, who had to live with all this bullshit growing up. But hey, everyone knew the difference between a vulva and vagina!

To my parents, for being such excellent pervs that I could only one-up them by going professional.

To my husband, who is super patient with me taking the fun out of every sexual topic by turning it inside out to examine the construction.

To everyone else I've ever dated or slept with … most of y'all were great examples of what *not* to do. Which is also helpful information, amirite? And to my best friend's exes, who are even more fun to dissect. Thanks y'all.

To the people who helped formulate so much of this book, including Edwin Tamayo, Aaron Sapp, Bonnie Scott, Susan Kaye, Maria Ballard, Amy Gonzalez and her amazing team at *The Love Shack Boutique* (where I am proud to serve as the official staff sexologist), and my dear friends/co-trainers from *The Center–Pride Center of San Antonio* (Naomi Brown, Robert Salcido, and Lauryn Ferris).

To my interns, who end up getting the weirdest supervision topics ever and put up with it.

And especially to my clients, who are brave as fuck in their healing journeys. Being part of your process is an honor.

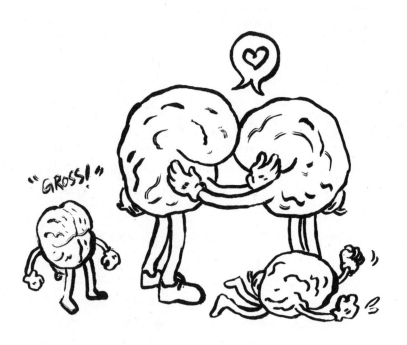

Unfuck Your Intimacy

USING SCIENCE FOR BETTER RELATIONSHIPS, SEX, & DATING

FAITH G. HARPER,
PhD, LPC-S, ACS, ACN

MICROCOSM PUBLISHING
Portland, Ore

UNFUCK YOUR INTIMACY
Using Science for Better Relationships, Sex, & Dating

Part of the 5 Minute Therapy Series
© Dr. Faith Harper, 2019
First edition © Microcosm Publishing, June 11, 2019
ISBN 978-1-62106-762-7
This is Microcosm #253
Edited by Elly Blue
Design by Joe Biel
Cover by Kelly Fry
Illustrations by Trista Vercher

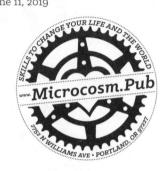

For a catalog, write or visit:
Microcosm Publishing
2752 N Williams Ave.
Portland, OR 97227
www.Microcosm.Pub

***To join the ranks of high-class stores that feature Microcosm titles, talk
to your rep:*** In the U.S. **Como** (Atlantic), **Fujii** (Midwest), **Book Travelers
West** (Pacific), **Turnaround** in Europe, **Manda/UTP** in Canada, **New
South** in Australia, and **GPS** in Asia, India, Africa, and South America.

If you bought this on Amazon, I'm so sorry because you could have gotten it
cheaper and supported a small, independent publisher at **Microcosm.Pub**

Global labor conditions are bad, and our roots in industrial Cleveland in the
70s and 80s made us appreciate the need to treat workers right. Therefore,
our books are MADE IN THE USA and printed on post-consumer paper.

Library of Congress Cataloging-in-Publication Data
Names: Harper, Faith G., author.
Title: Unfuck your intimacy : using science for better relationships, sex, &
    dating / Faith G. Harper, PhD, LPC-S, ACS, ACN.
Description: Portland, Oregon : Microcosm Publishing, [2019] | Includes
    bibliographical references and index.
Identifiers: LCCN 2018041764 | ISBN 9781621067627 (pbk. : alk. paper)
Subjects: LCSH: Intimacy (Psychology) | Man-woman relationships. | Couples. |
    Sex. | Dating (Social customs)
Classification: LCC BF575.I5 H368 2019 | DDC 158.2--dc23
LC record available at https://lccn.loc.gov/2018041764

Introduction

O k, intimacy. What the fuck do I mean by that? I mean, it's more than "just sex," right? In a nutshell, *intimacy is our human expression of our most important interpersonal (and yes, intrapersonal) connections.*

There are so many cultural messages about the "right" ways to experience intimacy and what is wrong, evil, sinful, or toxic. And about 99.44% of those messages are complete bullshit. Like, such down-to-the-brain-science-of-the-human-experience utter *bullshit* that I knew this was a topic I really needed to write about.

And creating and maintaining healthy relationships isn't easy. If it was, I wouldn't have a job, after all. We're all trying to figure this shit out. And the market bears that out, right? There are already tons of books out there about sex and relationships. My office and house are stacked to the brim with them. But most fall into one of two categories. They are either super straight-laced (presuming everyone is heterosexual, cisgender, married, Christian, middle-class, etc.) or they focus deeply on a very specific, niche topic like kink or polyamory.

And hey, a book specifically on sexual needle play does have its own target audience. *But where are the books for the rest of us?* I wrote this for people who don't fit the stereotype on *either* end. For those of us who are sex-positive (or are really trying to unpack our upbringing so we can be), open-minded (or want to be), non-traditional (no matter how we have tried to fit in with society's expectations), and seeking good information on the variety of issues that come up in our intimate lives.

Where is the inclusivity in mainstream relationship literature? The books that embrace all genders, all sexual orientations, all different kinds of relationship configurations, and all kinds of sexual interests? Seeing ourselves reflected in what we read is *fucking important*. Because we *all* have unanswered questions. Who and what do we like? How does trauma affect our relationships? What about our religious and spiritual upbringings? How do we unpack our own shit? How do we connect better with our partners? No matter your circumstances, you deserve a happy, healthy, active sex life if you want one.

My background is as a trauma therapist. In my work I've realized that one place trauma shows tends to show up is in intimate relationships. These are the relationships that require the most vulnerability and where we have the most to gain…therefore the most to lose. There are so many ways that sexual intimacy can get fucked up in, and because of, our current culture. I couldn't be a trauma therapist and *not* be a sex therapist. I've found myself working with people on issues surrounding their sexual relationships, so I started studying a lot. Enough, finally, to earn a postdoc in sexology.

Yes, this literally makes me a sexologist. My life does not suck with that as a job title. At my local coffee place my cup usually has "Dr. Perv" scribbled on it by the baristas.

As a therapist (ahem, sexologist), I think I have two main jobs. The first is coach: I help you figure out how to improve your performance. By performance, I mean reconnecting on an intimate level with yourself and your partners, present or future. Figuring out what is negotiable and what is not. Figuring out what you want your relationships to look like, and then starting to build in that direction.

The second job is intimately (see what I did there?) tied to the first: permission giver. I so often give people permission to start or stop doing things that can immediately impact their intimate relationships. If something is a problem, I give you permission to take it off the table; we can renegotiate it later. If there is something you want to explore, I give you permission to try it.

You are allowed to use a vibrator. You are allowed to stop intercourse if it hurts. You are allowed to schedule an actual date with your partner and enjoy each other's company. You are allowed to not go home for the holidays if sharing a bedroom with your partner is a point of contention with your family.

You can do the thing or not do the thing. My job is to help you figure out what the thing is and encourage you to get back out there and be in charge of your life.

I'll be right here, rooting for you!

What is This Book About?
This book is about building intimacy, with or without a partner, through personal and sexual expression. Especially through shit like consent, boundaries, and communication—which we don't talk about on the regular, although we really fucking should.

And this book is also about *sex*.

For most of us (and yes, I know this doesn't include my ace people... more on that later), sex is a big part of our lives and romantic relationships. It's not the foundation of a long term partnership, but it *is* that super-important spray insulation foam that fills in all the cracks and gaps, keeping the foundation airtight.

We can't separate the relationship stuff from the sex stuff, because *they are not separate issues.* Sex is generally an instrumental part of connection and communication between partners. So information on building, or rebuilding, that connection is here as well.

But wait! That's not all!!!! I'm not including a free set of Ginsu knives, *but* this book will also...

- Ask a lot of questions. It is surprising what we learn about ourselves when the right questions are asked.

- Apply to all types of relationships, not just heteronormative pairs. Many kinds of relationship configurations exist. Here is to honoring all of them.

- Acknowledge the impacts our upbringing, education, and sexual history have on our current intimate relationships.

- Address the impacts of all traumas in relationships: I am a trauma therapist first and foremost. Everything I have created over the years is intended to work *with* trauma recovery, rather than accidently trigger more trauma reactions.

- Address all the ways having a normal, human body can affect our sex lives. Medical problems, aging, having kids. All that normal, human stuff. Many of my referrals come from medical doctors, and I know these issues can be a big deal.

- Include some shorter-term strategies and tips for all the communication shenanigans and other everyday relationship shit that seems to, again and again, impact our sexual intimacy.

- Discuss all the ways we express sexual intimacy. Who we are attracted to and what we like to do with them when we get them naked.

- Attend to the really difficult work of repairing a relationship after there has been a break in trust.

- Help you realize that intimacy is serious business, without discussing it in a painfully serious manner. Life is tough enough, right?

Intimacy is one of the most fundamental expressions of who we are, because we define ourselves in relation to others. But life in general is better handled with as much humor as grace, and hopefully this book reflects that. Some of the stuff we do is empirically funny. And that is a damn good thing! I want to provide you a prescription to improve how you navigate intimacy and relationships. And I want you to giggle some while we do it.

There are some exercises in the book. Y'all have told me you really enjoy trying out the exercises I've included in previous books. Because once the science makes sense, the follow-up exercises don't seem like another dumb waste of time. We are going to just try some new stuff, if you are willing. This is a book of "let's try to figure out what's going on" *and* "here's some stuff that may help deal with it."

There is no 16-week plan here with steps and readings and assignments and all that jazz. This book is not a heavy, strategic relationship guide: Those already exist and there are plenty that are really good. If you're looking for a book like that, I work from and recommend a mash-up of relationship-specific therapies in my practice on any given day, and invoke strategies from Gary Chapman's *5 Love Languages*, Sue Johnson's *Attachment Theory*, and John and Julie Gottman's *Sound Relationship House Theory*, though I tend to queer them the fuck up (color you completely unsurprised).

This also is not a guide for either remaining in or leaving an abusive relationship: That is a whole other complicated endeavor that is way out of the scope of this book. If you are turning to this book because you trying to figure out if your particular relationship may be abusive, listen to your gut and seek some active help. There is no shame in therapy and other mental health support when you are going through some shit. So find someone with some training and perspective who can help you navigate your unique situation. It's really hard to see the forest when your face is pressed up against the tree's bark, right? I've included resources for people in abusive relationships in the appendix.

So just how is the knowledge here going to make your life better? Here's the plan: you are going to read this book and then go try some new stuff. At least, if this approach resonates with you. It's all up to you. These are just tools. You're the one who's gonna do the hard work. One of my favorite jokes is an old standard:

> "How many therapists does it take to change a light bulb?"
> "None! We encourage the light bulbs to change themselves!"

I know, groaner. But seriously, true. Have you ever tried to make a toddler who hates Brussels sprouts eat them? Not without sheer force, and the pushback ain't pretty. I can't make you do *anything* you don't want to do. Also, I'm not allowed by the regulations of my license to force you to do kegels. Aren't you relieved?

But I do know a lot about sexuality and intimacy work, and have found many common themes over the years. Many of these sections are based on columns written for different publications or my own blog, usually responding to questions people asked me. And if one person asks, they are probably not the only one wondering.

This book is divided into three parts.

Part One: How Our Intimacy Gets Fucked

Human beings are epically skilled at fucking up a good thing. How many bizarre messages have you received about sex and love over the years that really crimped your game? We've got shame issues, abuse issues, religious messages. That's a lot of shit to navigate.

Part Two: Unfucking Our Relationship with Ourselves

Have you never had a handle on what you want and who you are? Or did you once, and then everything changed because you changed? We certainly can't have the deep, interpersonal connections we want if we don't know what we actually, really want. That doesn't make us shitty human beings. It makes us products of a society that tells us how to be, what to be, and who to be. Which means many of us have work to do. What's our identity? How do we communicate with others? How can we interact with our own selves in order to be authentic, connected human beings?

Part Three: Unfucking Our Relationships with Others

Once we get a better handle on who we are, then we have to figure out who we are in connection with other people. And we need to learn to express that honestly, vulnerably, and all that horribly difficult shit. Remember, intimacy is interpersonal. Very few people are an island unto themselves. So how do we do this well in a world that is designed for us to fuck it up?

Getting Started

Sometimes (ok, a *lot* of times) we have stuff from our history that affects our current life and relationships. And sometimes (a *lot* of times) we aren't even aware of what that stuff is and where it comes from.

If you're experiencing challenges in your sexual relationships, many medical and therapeutic professionals will work with you on piecing together a "sexual history" of everything you've learned about sex and the kinds of sex you have engaged in. Originally this book was going to include a pretty intensive sexual history questionnaire. There was only one problem with that: *it's a pretty intensive questionnaire.* Completing such a form on your own has the potential of just being too much.

So instead, there are questions for reflection scattered throughout this book. But even scaled down, these might be anxiety-provoking. You do not have to answer anything that you are not comfortable exploring. You are not graded on completion here. It's totally and completely okay.

However, consider that any question that triggers a strong emotional response may be tied to issues in your current intimate relationships. And if things *are* getting stirred up, consider investing in your own self-care by working with someone who specializes in these issues. Yeah, I totally mean finding a therapist who specializes in this work. Ugh, I know. Not everyone needs to be in therapy, and it definitely doesn't need to be a long-term thing. But you deserve to be well and happy. And if you aren't getting there on your own, working with someone one-on-one is a worthwhile investment.

One of my favorite sayings is, "Crazy means doing the same thing over and over and expecting different results." So, let's try some different shit, okay?

Questions to Get You Started

- What was your reason for picking up this book? What's the one thing (or the main thing, or the biggest thing) you're hoping to get out of reading it?

- What negative experiences have you had regarding sex and intimacy? You don't have to write out a whole trauma narrative. Maybe just a word or phrase (e.g., "my chronic pain") or an identifier like "the abuse" for more intense experiences. It can be a good way to honor an experience without digging up everything about it in an untethered way.

- What messages have you received about sex in the past? Positive, negative, or neutral? Many people didn't receive negative messages per se, but it was simply omitted from conversations in your household growing up. Was sex discussed at all? If so, how?

- How was sex presented in the media you were exposed to when you were growing up? What kinds of stuff did you discuss with your friends and peers? With people you had romantic relationships with? How about now? Any differences?

- *If you could tell your younger self one thing about all these messages and experiences, what would it be?*

PART ONE:
How Our Intimacy Gets Fucked

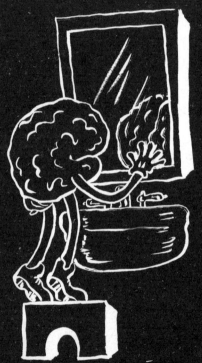

"You're doing a great job!"

Intimacy is *supposed* to be easy, right? I mean, neuroscience demonstrates that we are hardwired to connect to others. This is how we are supposed to *be*.

So if it's all so natural, why do we make such a fucking mess of it all the time? First of all, we're human and make mistakes because that's just part of the process. And it's an ever-changing process. We may have a handle on something and then, *boom!* Life thought it would be amusing to smash everything to smithereens. And as if *that* shit wasn't enough, there are so many toxic messages and mainstream bullshit shooting into our ear canals and eyeballs that we can't help but find our authenticity subverted on the regular.

There are a ton of issues that get in the way of fulfilling and healthy intimacy. I could write a fancy multi-volume leather-bound encyclopedia just on that. But for the purposes of this book, I'm gonna focus on the three that I see over and over again. The stuff that most of us bump into in some way, shape, or form in our lives. First up is trauma. Because trauma is a motherfucker that gloms its way into fucking up everything good we experience. Second is religion and spirituality. Connecting to something greater than ourselves is hugely important for a lot of people, but we can get inundated with interpretations and cross-talk that shame our experience rather than enhance it. And finally, we all struggle with bodies that age and change and sometimes require a new set of operating instructions. An aging body beats the alternative…but that doesn't mean we pay attention to our emerging needs the way we should be!

All our emotional work should start with figuring out what created the problem to begin with. I know that in my own life, understanding how I got somewhere is an essential part of getting out of it. I'm guessing you are also like that. I mean you're reading this right now, when you could be doing so many other things with your time, right?

Reading this book and doing the work serves two purposes. One is to become aware of the pitfalls that lead to your relational fuckery. But also, and I heard this over and over and over again from people who read my book *Unfuck Your Brain*, it's so helpful to know you aren't just fucking crazy. Or fundamentally broken. Or any of those things we tend to tell ourselves. Relationships get fucked-up because they are *hard*. Intimacy isn't easy shit to navigate. And everything we have ever been through (and that our partner(s) has been through) has been added to the mix. There is often a bunch of shit that has to be looked at and dealt with so we can get to the good stuff.

So let's start looking and dealing.

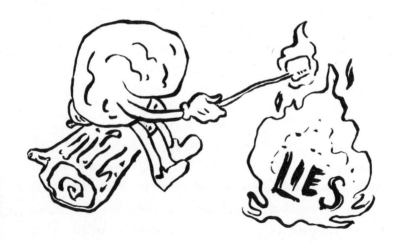

Five Myths About Intimacy

I wanna start with the basics. There is so much cultural mythology about what sex is and isn't that I'm going to be addressing over and over and over again within this book. But I bump into these five myths over and over again. I swear, if I could just banish these myths, everything else would fall into place. But then I wouldn't have a job and I'm not sure what else I would be capable of doing to save the world... I'll have to marinate on that one.

Myth One: Only Certain Types of Sex Are Real Sex

There is a ridiculous idea that certain types of sex are real. Or, at least, more valid and preferable to others. When we think of "real sex" we usually think partnered penetrative intercourse. But *do you know how many people have active and fulfilling sex lives and do not engage in partnered penetrative intercourse*? Or, for that matter, how many people have a lot of partnered, penetrative intercourse and still have epically miserable sex lives?

What actually *is* sex?

- A consensual act
- Between one or more people
- Involving the stimulation of the vagina, vulva, clitoris, penis, testicles, or anus

- For the purpose of pleasure and/or emotional or social connectedness.

Oral sex? Still sex. Solo sex? Still sex. There are not categories of sex that are superior to others. Unless the categories are good sex and bad sex. And you get to define those for yourself.

Myth Two: Sex Is Intuitive and Natural

We have this idea that sex should be spontaneous. And that we just sort of "get" what our partner wants. That we are going to run across a field of flowers in slow motion to each other. That everything should be free-flowing. And it will be amazing all the time forever with the right person.

Oh, please. What complete bullshit.

I can vouch with all my years of clinical experience (never mind all my years of, um, experience) that this kind of sex generally happens with people who are the worst possible matches, and in relationships that are completely unsustainable. Insecure attachments with ill-suited people cause a big chemical rush that's fun for a minute. But as most of us have learned the hard way, relationships like these mean you are hanging on for the ride as long as you can, but this ain't someone you bring home to momma.

Sustaining an enjoyable and long-lasting sex life with long term partners takes fucking *work*, y'all. And communication. And effort. And yes, calendar management. You don't pull together a huge Thanksgiving dinner for 20 people without any forethought, right? You make a plan. Making space for sexual intimacy is often also going to require some planning. Not having a slow-motion field of daisies experience doesn't mean your relationship is a sexual failure.

When I did my TedXSanAntonio talk "Sex, Shame, and Silence" back in 2013 (and go Google that shit if you haven't seen it, I'm still proud as fuck of it!) someone complained on Twitter that my definition of sex (the same one I used above) didn't include the word "natural." Now, sexual interest may be natural (unless you're asexual, demisexual, or graysexual, which by that definition would be unnatural), but how we have sex? *Not that natural.* We are constantly inventing ways to make it weird, interesting, complicated, and technologically advanced. Even professional pervs like the famous sex researcher Alfred Kinsey (who was known for tying up his nut sack with a cord and jamming a toothbrush up his dick) would be all, *"Damn, y'all,"* if he saw what we were up to now.

Sexual desire may be natural. But expecting sex itself to fit some category of natural means we are setting up ourselves for a lot of stigma and shame. Ain't nobody got time for that.

Myth Three: Sex Education Isn't a Universal Necessity
The US is the most sex-obsessed country that never talks about sex in pragmatic ways. It's everywhere. Every car ad is pervy AF. Your steak dinner? Sex was used to sell it in some way, shape or form. But sex education itself? Not acceptable. Just writing a sex column in the newspaper for the past three years has gotten me in hella trouble with the academic establishment. But if there is so much out there that isn't so natural and isn't so intuitive, then we need to have these conversations.

And you know who we need to have these conversations with? *Every-fucking-one.* Kids. Parents. People with intellectual disabilities. People with physical disabilities. People with severe chronic mental illness. Older people with changing bodies. LGB people. Trans folx. Poly peeps. Kinksters. We all need access to information about safe, healthy, and fun sex that meets our needs and desires.

Myth Four: Sex Is Not That Important In the Grand Scheme of Things
Ok, actually it isn't, *if everything is going well.*

If the sex is good, it's 10% of your relationship. If it's bad, it's like 90%. Is sex the most important thing in the world? Of course not. But people in Flint, Michigan still need clean water, and I bet they also still care about their sex lives and don't like it when things aren't going well.

Sex is important to most people. It's an important part of how we connect and communicate. And it often operates as the sparkly glitter-glue that helps keep relationships together.

If it's important to you, it's important. Don't let anyone diminish that.

Myth Five: Certain People Are Fundamentally Undesirable (and You Are Probably One of Them)

Thank you, media, for continuing to perpetuate the myth that there is only one kind of attractiveness and everyone else is just destined for misery and solitude.

Unless you're an epically unbearable asshole, there's someone out there for you. Your quirks and flaws (whether real or perceived) do not make you unworthy of great sex and wonderful love affairs.

I don't care how long you have been under the impression that you are an ugly duckling. I promise you that there are a decent number of people out there with a duck fetish. And there is nothing sexier than someone who loves their life and is out there enjoying it. That's how all us regular, flawed people find our partners. (Or on OKCupid. Semantics.)

My mission in life is to battle these myths in all the ways they show up in my clients' lives and in society. Kinsey was with me. We may have differing opinions about where a toothbrush goes (*FFS dude, in one's mouth*) but whatever. Opinions differ. Sex lives differ. And that's what makes it all so fascinating and fun. Everything contained in this book is a means to that end.

How Trauma Fucks Us Up

Trauma is an emotional response to a terrible event like an accident, rape or natural disaster. Immediately after the event, shock and denial are typical. Longer-term reactions include unpredictable emotions, flashbacks, strained relationships and even physical symptoms like headaches or nausea.

—American Psychological Association

So why are we talking about trauma? Besides the fact that, hi, I'm the trauma therapist who talks about trauma in relation to *everything*?

Actually, it's just that. Trauma *does* impact everything.

That's the reason I became increasingly interested in sexology as a field of study: The impact of trauma on people's intimate relationships was coming up over and over again and was often the impetus for people seeking support.

And for people who don't have Post-Traumatic Stress Disorder (PTSD) or some other kind of lasting trauma response? We all deal with situations that are *traumatic*. Things that shake us up and fundamentally change our lives in some way. And those changes have a huge impact on how we connect to others.

The *Diagnostic and Statistical Manual* (DSM) is the tool clinicians use to assign mental health diagnoses like PTSD. What they "allow" as trauma for a diagnosis is limited. I imagine any time you are trying to create a classification system you have to draw the line somewhere of what counts and what doesn't. But it's unfortunate.

Because so many life events that are not classified as a trauma by the DSM can cause a trauma response. It's not just the traditional stuff we think of, like being a soldier on deployment, being abused, or getting in a terrible car accident. For a lot of the things we talk about in this book, you may end up realizing they impacted you as a trauma. Fucked up messages you got about your body, your sexuality or gender not being respected by others, or being taught that the things you enjoy sexually are "wrong," "bad," or "inappropriate"—those can all be traumatic.

Of course not every trauma we experience causes a trauma response. A trauma response happens when our traumatic experience goes unresolved. Trauma becomes an issue when you notice an ongoing impact on your daily functioning. Which is just the clinical way of saying that your trauma history is impacting your ability to lead the life you want to lead. In short, we don't get what we need to heal. I wrote about this already (*Unfuck Your Brain*, Microcosm Publishing 2017), so I won't wax on too much about it, but a nutshell overview bears repeating.

How Does a Trauma Response or PTSD Develop?

We experience traumas throughout our lives. No matter how we try to protect ourselves, no matter how we try to remain safe, terrible things can happen. And sometimes, these terrible things happened when we were our youngest and most vulnerable selves—when we needed the protection of others who were unwilling or unable to provide that safety net.

Research shows that we are able to process and move on from many traumas on our own. We make sense of the events that have occurred and within a few months we regain our normal, baseline functioning. This may be a "new normal" that takes into account the impact of the trauma, but we are still able to navigate the world and our relationships in generally healthy ways.

But sometimes we get stuck. This usually happens within the first month of experiencing the trauma. For many, many reasons, either conscious or unconscious, we are not able to do the processing work necessary to make sense of the trauma and how it impacted our lives. This can often be for very pragmatic reasons. Processing a trauma can be a luxury of time and emotional energy that we don't always have. The brain may say, "we have other stuff to do right now, we don't have time to process a trauma." It could be that the traumas are coming in so fast and furious that our brains just go into survival mode and shut down processing to keep us safe. And sometimes our brains simply say "No. I'm sorry, I don't know how to make sense of this for you," and the processing shuts down.

These are the times where we develop a trauma response (or even PTSD). It may not be the biggest or the worst trauma we've experienced. But it is the one that, for whatever reason, we couldn't do the work on. And we begin avoiding the things that trigger the thoughts and feelings we haven't found a way to make peace with. And sometimes we have no idea that's what's going on.

A lot of times my clients are super aware that their trauma history is impacting their current relationships. They know there is work to be done and are actively doing that work.

Sometimes, however, we have no clue what's going on inside us and how it is affecting our relationships.

Story time, bear with me. Therapists love a good metaphor. My first car was a tiny, tin can of a thing with great gas mileage and crappy wiring. The taillight would go out on a regular basis, whenever a passenger accidentally kicked the wiring box. I was bopping along, thinking I had no problems when I was causing issues in traffic all around me. Fortunately, I lived in a small college town and knew most everyone. Someone would beep at me and yell *"Hey, Faith, light is out again! Almost rear ended you!"* And I'd pull over, wiggle the switch, and get it working again.

Why did I never know the brake light wire had been kicked out again? Well, I was in the car, driving the thing around. It seemed okay from my perspective—it was the people trying to navigate around me in our shared space on the road who saw the problem.

Fortunately, I never caused a horrible accident (or even a non-horrible one). Also, fortunately, other people were available to help me to recognize the problem and alert me to it.

Of course, trauma is rarely simple. Most people with a burned-out taillight aren't going to yell and argue, *"There is nothing wrong with my car! Go away!"* or even minimize, *"Yeah, whatever, I'll fix it later, it's not a big deal,"* as we are apt to do with an unrecognized trauma.

But this is a fantastic analogy about *perspective*. When we are going about our daily lives, we often don't see the broken bits that are so obvious to those around us. We are navigating our world, thinking everything is status quo until something or someone points it out to us. Or we crash.

Trauma and Intimacy

Intimacy, whether sexual or emotional, may trigger an unwanted response based on past traumas. You want to create a deeper connection with your partner and feel good inside your body, when something that you maybe didn't even realize was there becomes activated.

When I use the word trigger, I'm using in *clinically*. Meaning you stepped outside the present moment because something from your past made your brain say, "*Danger Will Robinson*" and freak out. The brain presumes that your past will be your future and goes into survival mode. Maybe you get flooded with memories. Maybe you freeze up and shut down. Maybe you completely disconnect. Your response is not about the present moment, instead your past experiences have gotten reactivated.

The thing I like best about the APA definition of trauma that opens this chapter is that it honors the fact that all types of traumas have the potential to affect our intimate relationships.

When I address with the impact of trauma on intimacy, most of the individuals I work with are sexual abuse survivors. But not everyone. All kinds of trauma can create a barrier to the intimacy we want and crave. This barrier can look like struggling to be in the present moment without being triggered, being unable to trust someone enough to be vulnerable, not knowing how to connect with a partner, not being able to identify and articulate boundaries, and feeling disconnected from your own body. Trauma is also associated with many other co-occurring issues including depression, anxiety, and addiction. Any or all of these things can also present obstacles to intimacy. Anyone who has ever been here is head-nodding right now.

What if There Was No Problem Before but It's Hitting Me Now. Why *Now*????

Congratulations, your brain feels safe enough to let you know that there is a problem and some work to be done. Doesn't that *suck*?

I have had many people tell me that their sex life with their partner was amazing at first. But as it grew deeper and more connected, they started having more issues. That sounds counterintuitive—the safer you are, the safer you should feel, right?

The more connected and emotionally attached you are to your partner, the scarier it can get. Being close to someone requires a level of vulnerability that you may fear will be taken advantage of. Trust is one of the hardest things for a trauma survivor to experience. But learning to trust again is an enormous sign of strength. Continuing to deepen your trust and connection can help you find the strength you need to continue your healing process.

Other life events can operate as a secondary trauma trigger, dragging you back to the initial unresolved event. Having a child together (whether through pregnancy, adoption, or fostering), or even just thinking about having a child together, can be a trigger. Moving away from a former circle of support can be another. Other big life changes, like in jobs, schools, or the relationship itself— living together, getting engaged, getting married—can also feel destabilizing, even when they are really good changes.

When someone comes to see me for trauma-related intimacy concerns that were not present earlier in the relationship, we usually find there is a fairly recent trigger that makes soooo much sense once we identify it. Oftentimes, just figuring that out is a huge part of moving forward. Because we all need to hear that what we are going through, and our reaction to it, is reasonable.

How Do I Unfuck My Trauma?

The excellent news is this: PTSD (and trauma reactions that don't meet PTSD diagnosis criteria) have the highest "cure" rate of any mental health diagnosis. Even complex traumas with messy co-occurring diagnoses are very, very treatable. The vast majority of people are able to recover from the symptoms they experience related to their trauma. Therapy works. I have zero problem saying in my out-loud voice that I go to therapy. There is zero shame in fighting for your own emotional health.

The important thing is recognizing that the trauma is the root of the other stuff going on, and will be the initial focus of treatment, providing what we now term trauma-informed care. Treatment is grounded in managing the trauma in a safe, structured way. If you are thinking about starting some therapeutic work related to a past trauma, consider finding a therapist trained in an evidence-based, trauma-informed care modality. But of course, different types of treatment are more effective based on your particular situation.

Use the types of interventions you feel comfortable with. I've had lots of patients who've announced, after being dragged to my office by a parent or family member, *"I'm not talking about that shit and you can't make me!"* And fair enough, getting better doesn't require you to unpack a trauma narrative. The important thing is to look for someone whose approach works for you. Ask them about their theoretical orientation, meaning how they approach healing, and find someone whose worldview aligns with your own.

I'm not referring just to traditional talk therapy. There is a ton of research behind somatic-based treatments like yoga, acupuncture, hypnotherapy, and the like. I recommend doing both somatic and talk therapy at once, but start with what feels safest for you and take it from there. There is no wrong way to start.

When considering what kind of treatment will work best for you, the question to ask yourself is *"What do I most need right now?"* No one knows more about what it is like to live inside your body and mind than you. What does your inner self say it needs? It could be

"I really need to tell this story," or it could be *"I don't even know how to be safe in my daily life right now."*

Listen to that voice. It's your survivor's voice, the one that has kept you safe during your trauma experience. It knows what you need to heal and move forward.

There are many ways to feel in charge of our lives again after our sense of safety has been violated. Self-compassion is a powerful way to take back your power after a trauma. I've included some self-compassion exercises at the beginning of Part Two of this book for you to check out. I have worked with people who became politically involved after a tragedy in an effort to change the social structures that allowed for the traumatic events to occur, people who began volunteering to work with others who have suffered similarly, and people who began engaging in new activities (such as boxing classes) and self-care (such as body work) in order to feel in control again. And one of the best tools I've found for helping people reconnect to intimacy after trauma is using sensate focus exercises with a partner, like the ones in Part Three.

Everyone's path to healing is different, but the common theme is a return to *empowerment* and *healthy coping in the present moment.* Figuring out what that might look like for you is the first step.

Some Questions to Ask Yourself
Empowerment

- What does empowerment look like to you? Feel like?

- How does empowerment connect to safety for you? Recovery?

- What are some ways you have experienced empowerment in the past?

- What are some activities you are interested in exploring to feel more empowered?

- What would be the first steps you'd need to take to explore these options?

- Is that something you are interested in doing right now? Why or why not?

Healthy Coping in the Present Moment

- What signs do you notice in yourself when you are triggered or activated, and not reacting to the present moment? What do you feel emotionally? Think? Feel in your body?

- When it comes to coping skills, we often already know what works for us, but it is difficult to remember to use those skills in the moment when we are distressed. What coping skills have worked for you in the past? What has been working lately? Which others are you willing to try?

- What can you do to help remember to use these skills? Are there individuals who can support you? Are there items you can have available (or items you need to get rid of!) in order to remain safe?

- What positive qualities did you develop in response to having to manage a traumatic life event? How could these skills help you in the future? This isn't an encouragement to gaslight yourself, by any means. While it is one of the hardest ways to learn a life lesson, many people have reported that dealing with a trauma did help them develop life skills that they didn't have before. Even if it was a lesson they never wanted to have to learn.

Creating a Trauma Response Safety Plan

Some individuals feel much safer if they have a very specific safety plan in place in the event of a trauma response. One of the most difficult things about being triggered is feeling so overwhelmed by the experience that making any decision about what to do in the heat of that moment feels impossible. Your brain isn't working the way it normally does, so having a plan to fall back on can be very helpful to both you and any partner with whom you feel safe in sharing that plan. Sharing your plan does not mean you need to share the entirety of your trauma history.

When we are sexually intimate, we are at our most vulnerable. Even if everything is going well, we can feel that we are stepping outside of our comfort zone. But this is the most important time for us to open lines of communication, especially if we feel unsafe. Many people create an effective verbal plan with their partner, meaning they just discuss what works for them via a conversation; others prefer the safety net of a more formal plan, like something written down, that you would refer to as needed.

You can use the following questions to outline a safety plan and open up the discussion with your partners.

- When you are feeling the most healthy, happy, joyful, and well what does life look like? How do you feel? How do you interact with others?

- What things do you do, or are you willing to start doing, as part of your daily wellness plan? What things have you noticed help you manage your triggers more effectively in a general sense? For example, many people have noticed that getting a certain amount of sleep and/or exercise is very beneficial to them. Some people feel better when they eat a certain way, meditate, pray, spend time with people they care about, or take time to enjoy hobbies that are meaningful to them. What activities do you think will work best in your wellness toolbox?

- What are some of the situations that you have come to realize are triggers for you? These are less the big catastrophic things that we sometimes worry about, but the smaller things that can happen on a more regular basis. For many people, this can be certain situations (like being in a crowded room or not doing well on a project), specific dates (like a holiday or birthday), or something they connect to in a very sensory way (like a certain smell or tone of voice). We often don't know what all of our triggers are, and may sometimes get triggered without any idea what caused it. But if we start keeping notes when it does happen, we can start to figure them out. So you may consider this list a work in progress that you keep adding to over time.

- What are your early warning signs that you may be getting triggered? What kinds of thoughts do you have? What emotions arise? What kind of behaviors do you engage in that you don't typically do?

- If you are triggered, what are the things you can do for yourself to help you manage your response? These are often things that you already do for your general wellness that become especially important in these situations. But they may also be coping skills or activities that you use when you are in especially tough situations.

- While there are a lot of things that you are able to do for yourself, there may be times you need help from others, especially if you are working on your intimate relationships. What do you need from others? Who do you trust to provide that support? How will you ask them about it?

- How will you know that you have been triggered past a point that you, and the individuals who typically support you, can handle?

- If you are at a point where you are not able to manage these triggers on your own, or with the assistance of the people who usually support you, what is the next step for you?

- Once your crisis has been managed, how will you know when you are feeling safe and secure again?

Once you try out your safety plan, jot down any notes about what worked and what didn't and make adjustments as needed.

Healing in Relationships

Whether you are just starting to explore a new relationship with someone or have been with your partner for a very long time, it is important to consider that they may be coping with an unresolved trauma. My late husband and I were married for ten years before he told me about his history of being sexually abused. It took him that long to feel safe with his story, and he was married to a therapist. It also made so many things that we struggled with make sense.

More often than not, statistically, any given person has experienced some kind of trauma. Cindy Crabb, who writes the beautiful and thoughtful *Doris* zines, suggests that you always assume anyone in your life has a sexual abuse history. This holds true for other traumas, as well. Cindy writes about how difficult it can be to discuss sex as a trauma survivor, especially if the trauma had sexual content. It isn't something we give much voice to in our society.

If you know or suspect your partner is coping with a trauma response, initiating the conversation rather than waiting for them to do so may be a very liberating experience. Of course, that doesn't mean forcing someone into a conversation, but offering it as an option can help you both walk through a door they didn't even know how to open.

Some things to try, or think about, if your partner has experienced a trauma or you think they may have:

- Expect them to not be present sometimes. Either during sex or just in general. If you get a sense that they are checked out, ask them if they are present. Ask if they need space to be alone, or if your presence helps. Ask what you can do to help if they are struggling. ("I think I lost you back there. Are you okay? Is there anything I can do to help?")

- Create a safe word. "No" is a crappy safe word, especially if you are into BDSM or edge play. Your word can be something silly that lightens the mood ("cheese doodles!"), or something that speaks to the experience ("darkness") but decide on this ahead of time with an action plan of what you will both do if the safe word is used during intimacy.

- If you partner needs space in the heat of the moment, offer them a chance to discuss it during a less stressful time within the next day or two. ("I know last night really triggered you, is there anything that you'd like to talk about now that you've had some time to think about it? Anything else that would help?")

- It's okay to ask. Did you fail your mind reading classes? I did. It's OK to say something like *"I get a sense that your mood shifted all of a sudden/It feels like you just shut down/Is something going on, I can't tell"* Try to do so in the most non-accusatory way possible, of course. But only ask once. A power struggle of "I'm fine!" versus "No, you are *not*!" is a terrible one that nobody wins.

- Be patient and understand that the sensations in a trauma survivor's body can be very contradictory. And the partner working through a trauma has to choose what sensations to focus on at each moment. That can be a complicated process for you to be present for. Sometimes your partner is doing everything possible to be okay. Maybe part of their healing experience is working through the issue in the moment and it's best to keep doing exactly what you were doing.

- Some things you can say include, *"I'm not sure if you liked that. I was hoping that you did and you said that you were okay, but I felt that maybe you were struggling. I want this to be good for you, so it won't hurt my feelings if there is something else you need or something you want me to do differently. And if you insist you really were okay, I promise to believe you until you tell me otherwise!"*

Remember that if your partner has a trauma history, they are the one who is responsible for themselves in the end. You can't rescue them or fix them. You can be part of their journey rather than an obstacle, but only if they let you and only if what they need is something you are able to give. This may be a continuing conversation throughout your relationship.

If you choose to be with them on their journey, don't forget your own wants, needs, and desires. Take responsibility for your self-care throughout the process, as well!

Grounding Exercises
Adding to your toolbox the coping skills that work best for you is good, proactive medicine. I've written a book entirely on coping skills (creatively titled: *Coping Skills*), which you can use to find a ton of ideas.

But the go-to skill I encourage everyone to learn is grounding exercises. And for a very specific, brain science-y reason. Remember when I said your brain expects that the past will be the future, so it operates accordingly? When we don't heal from trauma, our brains start *literally* reliving the experience when triggered. That's where grounding skills come in. The point of grounding is to refocus your attention on the present moment, so you can *stay here,* in the present moment, disrupting the *trigger-to-reexperiencing* cycle that so many of us struggle with.

There are three categories of grounding skills: mental grounding, physical grounding, and soothing grounding:

Mental grounding includes stuff like:

- Go over your schedule in your mind, or the steps it takes to complete an activity you do well. This accesses a different part of your brain than the one that's freaking out and helps you detach from the emotional memory being triggered

- Describe your surroundings in great detail. Colors, objects, sounds, smells. Give specific quantities (there are 37 books on that bookshelf, there are two chairs in the corner, etc.)

Physical grounding includes stuff like:

- Notice your breath. Just the physical in and out breathing experience. When your mind starts to wander, go back to the breath. You can also count your breaths. Or breathe in for four seconds and out for seven seconds.

- Touch objects around you and notice all the details of texture, pressure, heat, or cold.

Soothing grounding includes stuff like:

- Use a phrase or mantra that is soothing to you. It could be "I got this" or "This is temporary" or "I've survived 100% of the bullshit life has thrown at me thus far so statistics are in my favor that I will manage this fuckery, too." Whatever works for you.

- Picture a place that makes you feel safe. Zero in on all the details about that place. What does it look like, feel like, smell like? List details about the space to yourself.

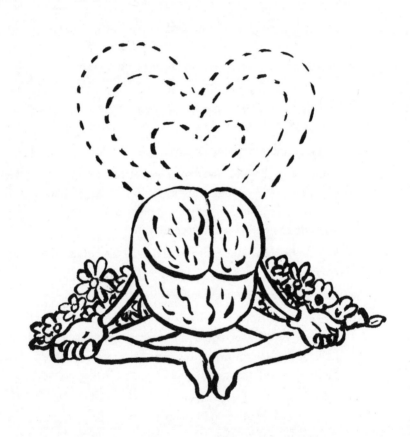

Sexuality, Religion, and Spirituality

They try to say what you are, spiritual or sexual?
They wonder about Solomon and all his wives.
In the body of the world, they say, there is a soul
and you are that.
But we have ways within each other
that will never be said by anyone.

—Mevlana Jelalu'ddin Rumi

Religion and spirituality are a big part of most people's lives. Even if they aren't part of your life now, chances are still pretty good that they played a huge part in the messages you got growing up, whether you wanted it or not.

I define spirituality as a larger experience of *purposeful belonging*. It can provide hope, healing, and connection to something larger than ourselves. Religion, at its best, is the organized expression of our spiritual selves. Just as we are hardwired for connection, intimacy, and touch, we are hardwired for ritual. For many people, religious practice fulfills their human need for the ritual expression of spirit.

The practice of spirituality, generally interpreted and defined within the scope of religion, has a history of seriously fucking people up. On one hand, we are told we are a beloved child of God (or another deity), and on the other we are told we are sinful and broken…that our thoughts, feelings, and behaviors bring shame to ourselves and those who love us. That's a good way to keep people in line, but it's a shitty way to help people create an authentic spiritual connection.

Being a spiritual person and expressing it through religious practice isn't wrong or unnecessary. But problems arise when aspects of that practice conflicts with something fundamental about *who we are as people*. Religion is totally boss when it reminds us to be good, and kind, and patient. To care for others who need caring for. But it's a huge fucking problem when it tells us our mere existence requires redemption.

I don't know *anyone* who hasn't had religious values from their past create some kind of internal conflict in how they express themselves as sexual beings. The first instance we generally think of is when individuals have a sexual orientation or gender identity that their religious practice deems sinful. And yeah, those are big ones. But in reality, conflicts between religion and sexuality occur in almost all of our interactions all of the time. What level of commitment should we have with another person before engaging in sexual activity—marriage only? Is solo sex acceptable or is that cheating on a partner? Is porn usage sinful? What about BDSM? Polyamory? Fetish play?

While I was raised in a deeply religious home, I was also fortunate enough to be raised by parents who attached no shame or restrictions to sex. Not everyone has had that experience, and many individuals struggle because of it. Most worrisome to me as a therapist is the enormous sense of shame that many people experience due to these conflicts. Brené Brown, the well-known shame researcher, notes that there is a fundamental difference between guilt and shame. Guilt implies that you made a mistake, shame implies that you *are* a mistake. Religious doctrine regularly invokes shame around sex and intimacy, with deliverance from this shame tethered to renunciation and confined behavior.

The general message you may have heard from sex-positive, affirming people is along the lines of *well then, fuck religion.* But not everyone wants to give up something that has grounded their identity in so many ways throughout their lives. It's akin to saying "Fuck your mom, she's an abusive asshole," and you're thinking, "Yeah, but she's still my *mom.* I dunno about that…"

The intent of unpacking your religious messages is not to dissuade you from any of them, but to help you recognize them and evaluate whether or not they make sense for your authentic self. Finding people you trust to help you work through the process as you reflect on these questions can be invaluable. Reading books by people who have dedicated their lives to resolving this conflict may also help… and if you are looking for good recommendations for books, check out the appendix!

Your mission here is to figure out what your unique experiences are in this domain and how they have been impacting your intimate relationships. Sometimes just asking the right question helps us go *"oh, yeah…I didn't even think about how that's a thing in my life"* So here's some shit to start asking yourself.

Some Questions to Ask Yourself

What is your spiritual and religious background?

- How have your spiritual or religious beliefs and practices changed through childhood, adolescence, and adulthood?

- Are your current religious or spiritual beliefs and practices different than many of the individuals who share your faith tradition?

- How do the teachings of your spiritual beliefs/practices address sexual intimacy? What role has it played in your spiritual development?

- Have you undergone any body modifications as a consequence of your religious beliefs that affect your sexual identity and practices (e.g., circumcision, castration, tattooing, piercing, or other body art)? If so, how have these changed your self-image? Your ability to engage in sexual intimacy?

How do you navigate your sexuality and spirituality now?

- How do you view the integration between your spiritual self and sexual self?

- Do your spiritual or religious beliefs and practices have any suggestions or rules about sex and intimacy? If so, what are your thoughts and feelings about these suggestions or rules?

- Do you engage in any sexual activities that are in conflict with these rules? If so, what are your thoughts and feelings about these conflicts?

- According to your spiritual or religious beliefs, what are the consequences of engaging in activities that are in conflict with this belief system? What are your thoughts and feelings about these possible consequences?

- Have you, or someone you know, experienced negative consequences from a conflict between your religious beliefs and your sexual practices (e.g. judgement, criticism, exclusion from certain events or membership in general, corporal punishment, etc.)? How has that affected you?

How do you negotiate spirituality in your relationships and community?

- If you are partnered, do you and your partner practice the same faith tradition? If no, how is your spirituality similar? How is it different?

- If you are partnered, do you or your partner experience any conflict between sexual expression and religious beliefs and practices? If so, how have these conflicts been negotiated? Have they been navigated successfully or are there still areas of tension?

- Have you received any guidance from a spiritual or religious leader about these conflicts? How about from a mental health or medical professional? What about family or peers? What was their advice or feedback? If you consulted with more than one person, did you receive conflicting feedback?

- Are there any areas that you and/or your partner feel are non-negotiable? Are there any avenues of compromise that you and/or your partner willing to consider?

- What are your thoughts and feelings about the intersection of spirituality and sexuality at this time? Have they changed from the past? Do you think they are likely to change over time?

- What would allow you to be both a spiritual and sexual individual?

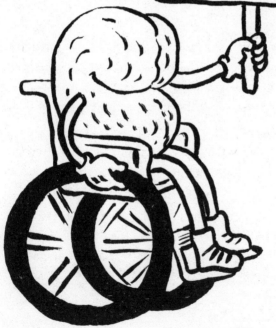

Changing Bodies and Other Fuckitude

Oh hey, there. I have a normal human body, capable of misfires and weirdness and continuing issues regarding its maintenance and functioning. I bet you do, too. In fact, I have a sneaking suspicion that we *all* do.

So why don't we talk about how this whole business of walking around in a wonky meatsuit affects our sexual intimacy? Because shame. Because embarrassment. Because not even realizing the connection between the two. Because not knowing what to say.

Trauma and societal messages aren't the only things that get in the way of having the sex life we desire. Maybe you struggle with chronic pain. Or you're otherwise healthy but broke your damn leg recently. Maybe you had a baby. Or you're just getting older, which does strange-ass shit to the body. It's time to start thinking and talking about these things in a better way.

Sexual Disorders

Keeping your sex life fully charged can be like tending a hothouse orchid. So many little things can go wrong and knock things off course. At some point in our lives for most everyone, we'll experience a sexual disorder.

The word "disorder" is a clinical term. A crappy one, I know. But it really only means that *things are not working in an orderly way.* And of course "orderly" is one of those consensus statements reflecting the general, cultural expectation of how things work, right? A disorder is not emblematic of being fundamentally broken or wrong or fucked up. It's just how it is sometimes. Which can add a layer of complication to our sexual intimacy. But we can totally work around all that stuff.

So let's start off by talking about the different categories of sexual "disorders" before we go into managing them, okay? We tend to think first of erectile dysfunction (because that's where the pharmaceutical dollars are), but there are actually *four* different types of sexual disorders.

- **Desire disorders** occur when there is no desire or interest in sex (this is not the same thing as being asexual ... which we'll talk about in Part Two).
- **Arousal disorders** happen when the mind is ready and willing (which doesn't happen in desire disorders) but the body isn't up to the task. This is the category for erectile dysfunction, though of course you don't have to have a penis to experience an arousal disorder.
- **Orgasm disorders** are what we call it when someone either cannot orgasm or it takes way longer and extra effort. This is also the category where "premature ejaculation" falls.
- **Pain disorders** are when intercourse literally hurts (this generally affects individuals with vaginas more than individuals with penises).

These issues may manifest in relation to other bodily changes, or they may present themselves *just because they do*. We are often so wrapped up in treating the symptoms by taking a pill (like the ones in commercials that involve some dude throwing a football through a tire swing) that we don't look at the underlying issues in a holistic way. Sex therapist and author Marty Klein states that this kind of work requires a different level of *sexual intelligence*. So let's ensmarten ourselves more on the topic.

Aging

Being in an aging body isn't anyone's idea of fun, but we all agree it beats the alternative. No matter how healthy we are, we all can benefit from attending to certain things in order to maintain a body that enjoys sexual intimacy.

The biggest sexual change most of us face as we age is hormonal. Testosterone and estrogen levels generally drop as we get older.

For cis men, this can mean erectile dysfunction or even just full arousal being more difficult to gain and maintain (read: a chubby instead of a stiffy). And when you do get the blood flowing, completing to orgasm doesn't always happen. Thanks, wang.

For cis women, the reduction in estrogen can lead to vaginal dryness as well as emotional and bodily changes that increase stress levels and decrease sexual desire.

There isn't a ton of research for non-cis folx on how any hormone therapy is affected by aging, but it is definitely something to take into consideration and chat with your doc about.

Disabilities and Chronic Disease

Of all the ways someone can achieve a "minority" status in the world, disability is the category where *any* of us can end up at *any* time. Whether you have a disability you've lived with your whole life or you entered this category later due to an accident or illness, it doesn't take a rocket scientist to realize that this can mean huge adjustments in all aspects of your life, including your sex life.

Some of the stuff that may come up around disabilities includes:

- Body image issues (your body may look and work differently than it has in the past, or than other people's around you)
- Anxiety about things changing or about things differing from what partners are used to or expect
- Anger at having a disability or chronic disease
- Feelings of guilt, as if the disease or disability is punishment for past actions
- Worry about a partner's unhappiness or dissatisfaction
- Worry about your partner being unfaithful or leaving you
- Frustration that your desire doesn't match your current access or ability
- Anger that your partner is healthy and you aren't

Possible issues for partners can include:

- Frustration with the limitations put upon your sex life because of the disability
- Feeling deprived. And angry about it. And then maybe guilty for being angry
- Resenting being in a caretaker role
- Guilty that you are not sick
- Challenged by your partner's changing body and struggling with physical attraction
- Worrying about hurting them

Of course, these kinds of feelings can come up for many other reasons too, but they are generally most prevalent when individuals are dealing with a chronic condition that seriously impacts their physical health and ability to express themselves sexually.

Childbirth

The general media portrayal is that birth is a mystical experience from which your body bounces back immediately. *Hah*. My kids are adults and I haven't gotten my body back.

Even if you had the most glorious pregnancy ever, with no morning sickness, stretch marks, or cramps. Even if you had the easiest birth experience ever, with no C-section, or episiotomy, or tearing, or hemorrhoids, and your body bounced right back? Childbirth still changes us. It changes our relationship with our body because we used it *to grow another human*. So many people have told me that during pregnancy and after birth their body simply didn't feel like theirs anymore, and it was a disconcerting realization.

And if you are breast or chest feeding? The whole matter of sustaining a small, dependent living thing with your body lives on. With chapped nipples, leaks, clogged, ducts, and all that other fun stuff. And hey, even if you aren't, you still have a tiny, fully dependent, and wildly fragile human attached to you on a regular basis. Your sleep is fucked. You are completely done with being touched by other humans by the end of the day. Talk about a disruption of an orderly sex life!

Other Mental and Physical Health Stuff

You might be thinking, *"Doc. I'm not in a wheelchair and I'm not 97 years old. This whole section doesn't apply to me."* But hey. We are all living in an increasingly toxic world and issues around sexual functioning are so damn commonplace for everyone that it merits discussion.

Mental and physical health diagnoses that do not *directly* affect sexual functioning can still *indirectly* affect it. Meaning, problems can occur because of something else you are living with. For example, over 100 million people in the United States have a diabetes diagnosis. Research shows that 50% of men and 35% of women with diabetes experience sexual dysfunction as a result. The good news is that if their diabetes is well controlled, those numbers drop quite a bit. The bad news is literally millions of people are struggling in this way and we aren't talking about it.

Cancer treatment, high blood pressure, heart disease, and just good ol' common stress can all impact our interest in sex and/or our ability to engage in the types of sex we want. And lest we forget, mental health also has a huge impact on the physical body. We talked about PTSD earlier, but all mental health issues impact our sense of self and our place in the world and that will absolutely affect how we connect to others. For example, if you are experiencing a depressive episode so bad you haven't had a shower in three days, the chances of you being interested in sex is probably about nil.

Long term medication use can also affect sexual functioning. This is by far not an exhaustive list, but just to give you an idea: hormones can cause desire disorders, anti-hypertensive (blood pressure) medications can cause arousal disorders, many antidepressants and some mood stabilizers can cause desire and arousal disorders. Even just plain old over the counter decongestants and antihistamines can cause arousal and ejaculation disorders.

So What Do We Do?

Everyone's experience is really unique, so I can't hook you up with a specific plan to have the best sex possible while dealing with physical changes, challenges, ailments, and disabilities. But I can help you look at some good general solutions, give you a list of questions to bring to your doctor's office, and then give you a few more things to think and talk to your partner about while you do this work.

Back in 2003 the medical journal American Family Physician published a piece on sexual functioning and chronic illness that had some pragmatic general advice about optimizing sexual functioning as much as possible for individuals with chronic issues. Here's the breakdown of what the authors of that article suggest, along with a few ideas from me. You'll notice that these are organized by intervention instead of by disorder. Disorders are just how issues manifest. They aren't causal in and of themselves. So any interventions we try should be about being as healthy as possible, not just popping one of those damn tire-swing pills.

Dietary Interventions

- No tobacco. No matter how you are getting it in your body. No smoking, vaping, chewing, etc.

- Limit your alcohol intake (if you're a drinker) and consider a no-drinking experiment to see if it makes a difference for you.

- Wait two hours after eating or drinking alcohol before engaging in sexual activity

- Eat as cleanly as possible. The fewer additives and toxins you consume, the better you'll feel in general. Cleaning up your diet isn't easy and it is expensive. I totally get that. But any small changes you can afford to make may have a huge impact on your wellbeing

- Consider whole food supplements to help you get the nutrients you are missing out on. For example, soil depletion means we have far less trace minerals in our fruits and vegetables than we did 100 years ago

- Talk to your doctor about what types of exercise you can tolerate physically. Match that list against your list of exercise you can tolerate emotionally. Gentle movement that actually feels good can be incredibly beneficial in building strength and flexibility … or at least slowing the loss of strength and flexibility

Medication Interventions

- If you have chronic pain, take your pain medications 30 minutes before starting sexual activity

- Talk to your prescriber about which of your medications may have sexual side effects and discuss replacing them with something you tolerate better or finding ways to manage those side effects

- Consider complementary therapies like acupuncture, neurofeedback, biofeedback, and the like to help manage pain

- If your diagnosis has caused an onset of depression (which is entirely probable and makes a ton of sense), make sure you get that depression treated

Environmental Interventions

- Keep your home at a comfortable temperature. If you need it warmer to help your pain, do that. If you need it cooler to help your breathing, do that. Figure out your best operational setting for sexual intimacy and adjust as needed

- Plan sexual activity for the times you know you have gotten the most rest and your energy levels are good. This may be time of day, time of week, or time of month. For example, many people on chemotherapy get breaks in the cycles and know their energy levels are the best near the end of the break

- Be flexible with types of sex as well as bodily positions. Use pillows, wedges, or other supports if they help

- Consider using sexual aids (sex toys!) to augment your experience

Emotional Interventions

- Communicate openly and honestly with your partners about your needs, wants, likes, and dislikes

- Explore your own body through solo sex. It's easier to communicate what works for you if you've already figured it out for yourself. Plus regular orgasms may help you feel better physically and emotionally

- Use intimate touching that isn't designed to lead directly to sex every time

- Use all of your senses to focus on the parts of your body where you enjoy stimulation the most, even if they aren't traditional erogenous zones. A friend of mine sustained a nasty spinal injury. He recovered fully, except afterwards he realized that he had more sensation above the point of injury than below. While he is still able to maintain an erection, his neck being stroked was the best way to encourage his arousal.

Questions For Your Doctor

In a perfect world, your doctors would be the ones opening up conversations about sex, saying something like, "It's pretty common for people with this condition to notice that it's affected their sex lives in some way. Have you noticed anything we need to address?" This opens the door for you to bring up any questions you have. However, a lot of doctors are uncomfortable bringing up the topic of sex, even if they are comfortable discussing it. For example, many docs could tell you that kegel exercises can help you better control your PC muscles, which can help with bladder control, premature ejaculation, and pain associated with penetration. But they'll only talk about this if you bring it up.

So you may have to be the person to say you have questions. And if they can't answer the questions, tell them to refer you to someone who can.

Not sure what to ask? Here are some questions to start with:

- Are certain kinds of sexual activity off limits? Which ones?

- What is the safest kind of sexual activity for me right now?

- What should I do if I have pain or medical issues during sexual activity?

- Will my meds affect my sex life (libido/desire/ability to perform)?

- If so, do I have other medication options? Other ways of managing these effects?

- Are there any circumstances under which I should avoid sexual activity?

- Will I ever be able to [fill in the blank] again? What are the best case, worst case, and most likely scenarios?

- Is it possible I could regain the ability to engage in some sexual activity that I can't do now? What would help me be able to do that?

- Are there any resources that are specific to my situation that you recommend?

- Are there any other treatment professionals you recommend me working with that may help with this issue?

Questions For Yourself

When it comes down to it, self-reflection and partner communication may help far more than any other doctor or sex therapist. Here are some things to think and talk about.

- What was the quality of the sexual relationship before the illness/injury if you had one? Sometimes if things were already not going well, a new health issue can become the excuse to just stop trying altogether.

- What makes something "sex?" Has that changed? Could it change to encompass more activities than you've done in the past?

- Where do you feel sensation and pleasure?

- What do you miss most?

- What does your partner say that they miss most?

- What things are working well?

- What do you most want to communicate to your partner?

- What are your fears in doing so?

Kegel Exercises

Being healthy is far easier if we exercise, right? Sexual health has its own exercise...the Kegel. Obviously, Kegels aren't magically curative for all kinds of sexual disorders but they are one of the go-to exercises that really help a lot of people! Kegel exercises are designed to strengthen the pelvic floor muscles, focusing specifically on the "PC" (pubococcygeus) muscles. Kegels have tons of practical use for all kinds of issues, whether you have a vagina or penis.

Dr. Arnold Kegel was a gynecologist who developed these exercises for women who had pelvic floor weakening post childbirth. He found another interesting side benefit: His patients who were doing kegels regularly were achieving orgasm with greater ease and frequency, and had a more intense experience, showing that kegels have an additional benefit to sexual intimacy. They have been found to help both women and men better achieve orgasm, and can help both sexes feel more in control of their sexual experience for a few reasons:

- Kegels help control urinary incontinence, so many individuals feel more secure during sexual activity and less likely to leak urine.

- Kegels help give the individual on the receiving end of penetrative intercourse more control over the experience and more intense orgasms. They also create a tighter vagina or anus, therefore increasing the pleasure of the penetrating partner as well.

- Kegels help bring more blood flow to the pelvic region in women and the perineum region in men, potentially intensifying your arousal.

Kegels can be done with or without an aid (such as a dildo, vibrator, or tool designed specifically for kegel mastery like Betty Dodson's kegelciser). They can be done solo (which is usually a good place to start) as well as during penetrative intercourse (which can be a *lot* of fun for both partners).

Here's how to do them:

- Locate the muscle group in question by squeezing the muscles you use to stop your urine flow. If you are urinating and are able to halt the flow, you have the right muscle group. Your stomach and buttocks muscles should not tighten in the process. You also don't want to do your kegel exercises when emptying your bladder on a regular basis. That can lead to weakening the pelvic floor muscles which can prevent you from fully emptying your bladder (which, in turn, can lead to an increase in urinary tract infections).

- If you are using a kegel aid, lubricate the aid before insertion and practice kegels lying down. If you are not using an aid, it may be of benefit at first to practice lying down.

- Squeeze the muscle group for three seconds, then release for three seconds. Complete 10 to 15 cycles of squeeze and release.

- Try to do this at least three times a day. The more regularly you perform the exercise, the better results you will get (just like any exercise).

As you get more comfortable doing this, you will find that you don't have to set aside "kegel time" to be effective. You can do them while engaging in other activities since no one will know what you are up to—unless of course you are doing them during sex, in which case your partner will know and appreciate it!

PART TWO:
Unfuck Your
Relationship
with Yourself

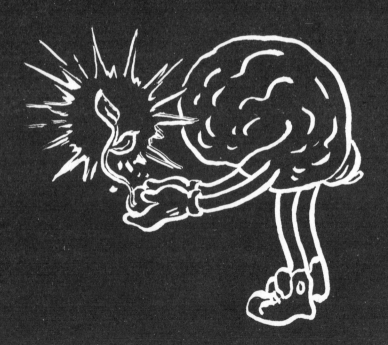

I f you are reading this right now, you are a grown-ass human (either officially grown or grown enough to know what you're reading) who understands that the only person you have any real power over is yourself. Sucks, doesn't it?

That's why we are starting by dealing with our own shit first. After we get a better handle on where some of our more fucked up messages about intimacy come from, the best place to get to work is with the person we know the best, have known the longest, and are gonna be stuck with forever. Which is to say, our own damn selves. When we do our own work, understand our own responses, and stay truly connected to our own bodies, we are far better able to connect with others.

Much of this part of the book is focused on your experience of your body. Super weird in a book about relationships with others, right? Why don't we just move on to the partner stuff, FFS? Because our relationship to our own bodies is an essential starting place. How can we know who we are in relation to others if we have no idea what's going on within ourselves? We really can't separate the body and mind, though we sure as fuck keep getting that as a message!

We'll start with with ways we relate to our bodies emotionally, like being self-compassionate and figuring out our boundaries. Then we'll move on to how we live in them physically. Which means, yes, totally going to talk about body image and masturbation.

It's entirely okay (and really very normal) if everything you read in this section is super new to you. Or if it's stuff you've tried but felt like you failed at accomplishing. You may be fighting years of conditioning around sexual expression, and that may take awhile. Keep fighting for yourself. You have every right to be empowered, comfortable in your skin, and deeply satisfied with yourself!

Self-Compassion

Self-compassion is a mindful awareness of your value and worth as a human being. A human being who is flawed, imperfect, and struggling.

This is opposed to self-esteem, which is based on external events. Self-esteem crashes when we are unsuccessful, either by the standards of others or ourselves. Self-compassion, on the other hand, is inclusive instead of competitive. It is always available to us, even when we are not our best selves or successful by the standards we have established. And it's pretty much impossible to connect with others intimately if we don't have some level of comfort with our own flawed existence.

I think of self-compassion as a *gift of desperation*. Meaning, it's something that we come to when we are desperate enough to stop trying to do things the way we always have and try something completely different. Self-compassion was a huge struggle for me when I first learned about it in my mid-30s. Beating myself up wasn't working. Willing my self-esteem to be magically better didn't work either. Finally, I was desperate and exhausted enough to just try loving myself instead. And my whole fucking world changed.

Why is self-compassion so hard? We are raised with the socio-cultural message that we are responsible for our own actions. That's not a bad thing, and to a certain extent I'd say it's an empirical truth. However, tied to that idea is a belief that you should never let yourself off the hook for failings and bad behavior. And because we all fail frequently, repeatedly, and epically, because we are imperfect, we are always bashing ourselves against the metaphorical rocks.

That voice inside your head? The one that tells you that you must be perfect?

That voice is setting you up for failure.

However, self-compassion is *not* the same as letting ourselves off the hook. It does not mean we lower our standards, throw huge pity parties for ourselves, or indulge in continuous bad behavior. It means we give ourselves the same support, encouragement, and tough love that we would give to our dearest friends and family. It is the mediating voice between self-criticism and self-complacency.

As human beings, we are flawed and fault-filled. We also have the ability to accomplish amazing things and have deep, fulfilling relationships. When we view ourselves with compassion, we see the truest picture of both our flaws and our capacity for transcendence. And when we value ourselves for our efforts, we learn to confront, forgive, and transform our shortcomings.

Intimacy work can be fun, but it is quite often difficult and requires confronting issues and having conversations that we are not used to. Our ability to face many of the barriers to intimacy requires a great deal of self-compassion: it is the currency we need for change. One of the truest forms of emotional intelligence, it means we are both mindful of and engaged with our thoughts and feelings. Life, in general, requires a great deal of self-compassion. And the more we connect to our own failings, the more we are able to empathize with the failings of those around us. Compassion starts at home then radiates outwards, right? Holy shit, that sounded woo-woo as fuck. Truth, tho.

Kristin Neff, who literally wrote the book *Self-Compassion*, breaks this sort of work down into three parts. My version adds a fourth component (self-empathy) as a way of focusing in on your core experience during the process. My hacked model is as follows:

- **Mindfulness**—Here, this simply means awareness of our current experience. Literally what is going on inside you in the present moment—all of your thoughts, feelings, and physical sensations. Without trying to suppress it or control it or judge it. Just saying "Oh hey. There you are."

- **Self-Empathy**—Self-empathy is thoughtful and active listening to our feelings, thoughts, and sensations. The same way you would listen to a friend. This term comes from psychologist and mediator Marshall Rosenberg's work on non-violent communication. With mindfulness, we are tuning in to all of our internal experiences. Self-empathy, per Rosenberg, is an inner questioning of the core inner experience to which we are the most attuned. What do you notice most? What is most important to you?

- **Self-Kindness**—This means being tender with ourselves rather than shitty and judgmental about our failings. Similar to the practice of loving-kindness, which is a consideration of and tenderness toward others, compassionate self-kindness means actively giving ourselves care and comfort in the presence of our own pain. If you cut your hand, even doing something dumb, you would go clean it off and bandage it, right? We do this with our physical selves, but rarely with our emotional selves. Self-kindness is the cleaning and caring of the wound, so it can heal.

- **Common Humanity—**Recognizing our common humanity means simply, recognizing "wow yeah, I'm human, and I'm hurting, and other people feel this way too...we're all part of it." It's the realization that I am not alone in my pain and imperfection, and do not have to isolate myself while going through it. I am experiencing something that all human beings experience because we are all fucking human.

Self-compassion is something I hope you will explore holding for yourself throughout this unfuckening process. Intimacy is so very raw and reaches in to the core components of who we are individually and in connection. This process is replete with opportunities to practice self-compassion. And, honestly, will probably be the thing that most helps you through it.

As you move forward through this book, you are going to bump into all your intimacy hobgoblins. These are the perfect times to practice self-compassion. Body issues? Bullshit religious messages? A history of fucked up relationships? Are you used to beating yourself up, and then beating yourself up for beating yourself up? Aren't you really fucking sick of it? Gift of desperation time.

Questions to Ask Yourself

- How do you deal with making mistakes? With "failing" or being "a failure?" How badly does it fuck you up? Do you ruminate and perseverate and tell yourself horrible fucking things?
- How does your self-criticism impact your internal life and choices? How does it affect your relationships with others?

- Where is your best opportunity for growth right now in your relationship with yourself? What do you want to change? What scares the fuck out of you about trying to do so?

Some Self-Compassion Exercises to Try:

- Approach your emotions with curiosity rather than judgment. Just notice them instead of labeling them in a positive or negative category. As in "Oh, I'm feeling …. I wonder where that is coming from? I wonder what that's about? Is that emotion connected to something I need that I'm not getting?"

- Reflect back on a time when someone you cared about was going through a difficult experience. How did you support them? They may have fucked up royally, but you still recognized their personhood, right? Now, how can you use those same skills for yourself?

- Picture someone who is a kind and encouraging motivator for you. If you don't have any ideas on deck, picture me. I totally want you out there doing awesome shit and having a fulfilling life. What motivation strategies would this person use to help you move toward change? How would they approach you? Guess what: now you have to do this for *yourself*!

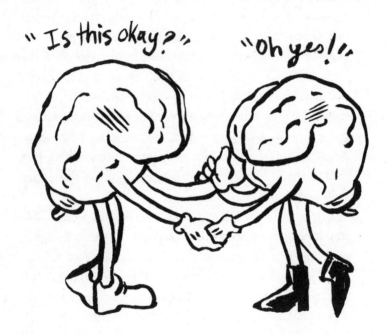

Boundaries

Nutshell definition? Boundaries are *the everyday expression of consent.*

Boundaries within an intimate relationship can take many forms. They range from sexual boundaries (*"No butt stuff, stop pressuring me!"*) to privacy boundaries (*"Stay out of my journal, FFS!"*) to just everyday interactions (*"I don't like to be touched when I'm cooking"* or *"I need 20 minutes to decompress when I get home from work"*).

Boundaries help us feel safer and more secure in a world that is usually anything but. They are our foundational supports for existence. Having healthy boundaries means understanding where we need space and where we need scaffolding and communicating those needs to the people around us. Boundaries are necessary in all of our relationships, but they are the most important in our intimate relationships. And it's one of the great ironies of the human condition that our closest relationships are the ones in which our boundaries are often the least respected.

Boundary-setting in relationships is rarely overt and action-oriented. Instead, in modern culture, and especially around sex and intimacy, boundaries are more often defined by a lack of words or action. Not talking about things sends the message that these things *aren't worth talking about.* That they don't matter. That what we want, need, and desire doesn't matter. That who we are in relation to others doesn't matter. And that seeps into *all* our other interactions.

If boundaries are a relational foundation, and you realize that the foundation needs some work, putting in these support beams now may help prevent a catastrophe later.

So where do we start setting positive, healthy boundaries? Boundaries are inherently unique to each person and there is no one-size-fits-all way to manage them. But we can create a framework for discussion. We can look at ourselves and start conversations that we haven't had before. And this has the power to create huge shifts not just in our lives, but within the rest of the world.

What Are Your Boundaries?

Understanding your boundaries is the first step in communicating them. And hey, don't forget there is a whole chapter on unfucking your communication later on in this book. But you gotta know *what* to communicate first, right?

Here are some essential questions to consider for yourself within your intimate relationships.

- What's your deal breaker?

- What is the absolute no fly zone in your intimate life?

- When do you know you are done with an intimate partner or situation for good?

Okay, do you have an answer? Now it's gut check time.

- When you read those questions, what was your *emotional* response? Not what you *think* you should have answered, not what you know the intellectual answer to be, but what your *body* tells you the answer actually is.

This is where we listen to, and within, ourselves and pay attention to the answers we find. It's totally okay if you have stuff bubble up that surprises the shit out of you. Or if you feel completely panicked because you have zero clue as to what your answer is. That's totally OK, friend. And utterly to be expected in a culture where we hear *"Hey, boundaries are a big thing, what's important to you?"* as we grow up.

Unless you're a cat (*"Touch one of my toe beans and I will end you"*), you probably have had some struggles in this area. We work through it by paying attention to our gut reactions and longer-term responses to how people interact with us. Explore this topic. Ask people you trust to weigh in (your awesome friends, your rock star therapist, etc) and see how your body resonates.

How Strict Are Your Boundaries?

Boundaries can be rigid, permeable, or flexible. *Rigid* means nothing gets through, ever, and there is zero space for negotiation. *Permeable* means that everything gets through if it wants to. Your boundaries are defined for you, but attacks come from the outside, and you don't know how to hold your ground. *Flexible* boundaries, on the other hand, come from the inside. Where *you* are the one willing to compromise in certain areas, because it may lead to the betterment of the relationship and emotional growth for yourself.

Some boundaries should be rigid, if they defend real safety and security. These are the boundaries that reflect needs rather than wants. Some boundaries in that regard are universal. Most are not. Boundaries that are rigid for me may not be an issue at all for someone else. Someone who is neurodiverse may need more alone time than other people. Someone with a trauma history may never feel comfortable with certain sexual positions. We have all had different experiences and have different needs based on them. That's part of the human condition. Our boundaries also change in different relationships, different circumstances, and different points in our lives.

And honestly, being a rigid asshole is just as bad in the long run as letting someone stomp all over our boundaries. With all boundaries, we need the capacity to negotiate while still maintaining our safety and not becoming a total pushover. It's that nebulous, hard-to-define difference between flexibility and permeability. For example, when you're exploring intimate touch with your partner, maybe certain areas of your body are off-limits right now (a rigid boundary) but at some later point you might be willing to try it if the lighting is adjusted and a timer is set (a more flexible boundary).

Here are some questions to explore your existing boundaries (whether or not you've started communicating them to others):

- What messages have you internalized about your right to healthy boundaries and the ownership of your individual needs?

- Generally speaking, are the majority of your boundaries rigid, flexible, or permeable?

- Which of your boundaries are rigid right now? Are there any that need to be challenged in that regard? Are there any that need to be more rigid?

- Which of your boundaries are permeable right now? Are there any that need to be challenged and strengthened into being flexible or even rigid? Do you have any boundaries that should remain permeable? If so, how does that permeability support, sustain, or serve you at this point in your life?

- What would your ideal boundary balance look like? How close to this ideal are you right now?

- What is something that is actively in your control that you can work on to move in the direction of your ideal?

How Do the People in Your Life Respond to Your Boundaries?

Boundaries are fundamentally relational. If you hermit it up by yourself far from society, you won't need boundaries.

If you are struggling with the questions above, this can be a really good perspective-gaining section for you to work through. Because we're looking for patterns here, right? So these are really important questions:

- Which people in your life respect the boundaries that you effectively communicate? What do these people have in common?

- Which people do not? What do these people have in common?

If, generally speaking, most people in most situations don't respect your boundaries, then it's time to look at how you are communicating them. Maybe you aren't expressing them as effectively as you thought. Guess what? There may or may not be an app for that, but there is *definitely* a chapter in this book for that. So yaaay…help is on the way!

But if you are struggling more in specific relationships or with specific people who keep blowing past your boundaries, then you might, in fact, be dealing with an asshole, or an asshole-infused situation, like a really shitty office culture.

Before you apply some smackdown, and especially if you're looking at a newer relationship, consider a few other possibilities for why your boundaries aren't being respected:

- The possibility that this person has other stuff going on, such as medical or emotional health issues, that make attending to what you communicate difficult for them.

- The possibility that this person is on the autism spectrum, making traditional conversation cues difficult for them to suss out.

- Maybe the individual is neurodiverse in other ways (eg, ADHD) and has a hard time attending to relational, non-verbal signals and implicit messages.

- The possibility that this person is an abuse groomer digging in their heels in an attempt to get you under their emotional control.

If the last scenario is the case, you know what you need to do. Seriously, get yourself safe. If the other scenarios are a possibility, it's time to have a different conversation. Ask the person how they respond and learn best and try adapting your communication style. Chances are that within the first three scenarios, you will need to take away any need for guesswork by expressing your expectations as concretely as pavement. Ask for their attention, express yourself clearly and directly, and elicit feedback regarding their understanding.

You may be in a situation where you just have to suck it up, too. I'm well aware. You have a shitty job you can't afford to leave. Or you have a shitty family that you can't, at this time, extract yourself from. You have to weigh your options before deciding to throw down over a boundary.

This is another place where the flexibility thing comes in. You will find tolerating a lack of respect of your boundaries *far* easier to manage when you acknowledge that you are making a choice to maintain the relationship rather than maintain the boundary. It may be the best choice for you at this moment. Remind yourself that this epic dickitude is just slightly better than the alternative, so you are choosing to accept it for right now. This perspective can really help you tolerate how upset and angry you feel. It may also propel you into creating the action plan you need to extract yourself from an increasingly shitty situation, rather than sitting in that slimepool of disrespect and disregard forever.

Stuck with motherfuckers who push every last button? One of the tricks I've found that has really helped me with those kinds of assholes is to imagine a clear pane of glass between me and them. I can hear and see them (because, hey, we are talking about the people we literally can't avoid, right?) but their emotional bullshit stops at the glass. This is especially helpful for us Counselor Troi empath-type people. We can respond to the content of their words and actions without being emotionally drained by whatever awful, negative, or manipulative forces are driving them.

How Do You Respect Other People's Boundaries?

Ok, so now that we have a better idea of your own boundaries... That was a fuck-ton of emotional work, wasn't it? Ugh, yeah. Let's go ahead and finish off the navel-gazing by looking at how you respond to the boundaries of others.

- Generally speaking, do people tend to respond positively to you? Do they tell you they feel comfortable sharing with you? That you hear them without judgment?

- Do you have people (or at least one person) in your life with whom you are able to have deep and authentic exchanges of ideas and feelings?

- Are you able to maintain these relationships over a long period of time?

- What kinds of situations make it hard for you to respect the boundaries of others? Is it with certain people? Or when people are making certain decisions that cause you concern?

The first three questions are a good self-examination of whether or not you are able to maintain relationships. If you struggle with the boundaries of others, it will start to eat away at your relationships in general. Let's be honest. Do you know anyone who is bad at boundaries but somehow still maintains healthy relationships? I don't.

If you read the first three questions and had an "Oh, *fuck*" moment, that doesn't mean you should put down the book and immediately start emotionally self-flagellating, okay? We generally learn good or bad boundary setting from those around us. If no one modeled healthy boundaries for you in the past, how were you supposed to learn? And since no one is handed the boundaries manual at birth, a lot of us have to figure it out later. As you start being mindful of boundaries in your interactions, I bet you will see serious, positive changes in your relationships overall.

The fourth question is more universal. Because I *promise* we all have situations where we struggle to respect other people's boundaries. It might be with family members you care about, when you see a friend making the same dumb decision for the 97th time, or when you see someone engage in a behavior that you've previously seen lead to a bad end for yourself or others. Those kinds of situations can really make it hard to respect their boundaries.

And it's okay to communicate that. To say something in the vein of:

I'm having a hard time respecting your boundaries right now because I'm really worried about you. I don't want to start bossing you into doing what I want you to do. It might be better if we don't discuss this particular issue because I can't really be impartial.

That's a nice way of saying, "I don't agree with your decision but I support your ability to make it for yourself. I may need to step away from the situation to maintain that support, but that's about me... not about you." It's the nicest way I can think of it to avoid a *"They're gross! Break up with them!"* conversation that's only going to get you into trouble.

It's also okay to ask for clarification on what level of support someone is looking for. I struggle with the boundaries of my adult kiddos. Makes total sense, right? I still want to parent them. When they ask for me advice, I ask straight out: *Do you want the mom answer or the supportive-adult-in-your-life answer?* This gives them the opportunity to let me know how flexible their boundaries are about my interference in the situation. And has probably saved us from any number of fights over the years.

I know. I know. This is ridiculously difficult. This learning-boundaries thing that no one ever taught you in the past. And you may find that people hardcore fight you on it when you start setting new limits.

And that may mean you have to make some difficult choices. Because when it comes down to it, we either let the world dictate our boundaries for us *or* we communicate them with what we do and say. As off-kilter as it can be at times, I would *far* rather experience the discomfort of difficult conversations than let the world determine what is going to happen to me.

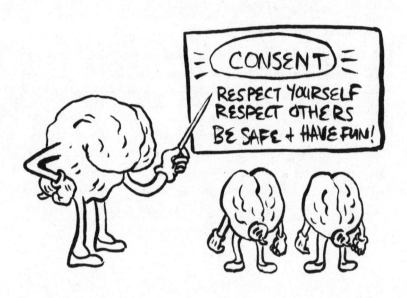

The Consent Commandments

Consent is an active process of communication. It's not just the *"can I [blank] this part of your body with [blank] part of my body"* that we see repeated ad nauseum in mainstream media. It's just as much my cat flattening her ears when she doesn't want pickie-uppies. Or my husband scrunching his face when I even *think* about putting onions in whatever I'm cooking.

At its core, consent is simply *permission for something to happen*. Consent defines our rules of engagement, the ones we express through boundaries.

We have all had experiences where our boundaries were violated and others did not request permission to interact with us, especially in regard to sex and intimacy. I am continuously surprised/not surprised by how often my fellow clinicians in the field, even, misunderstand the need for active consent in relationships. We presume that permission for one activity implies permission for others.

Consent provides a safe framework for interactions. For those of us with trauma histories, a safe framework can be a very healing experience. And, equally important, it allows us to experience own our desires in a sex-positive way. In an ideal situation, you aren't having to be convinced, you're saying *yes*!

These ten commandments came from a class I was teaching a few years ago for clinicians working with teens. We walked through group activities they could use to teach consent and boundaries *and* work with issues related to boundary violations. When it comes down to the basics, however, there are some fundamentals that apply universally. And as a good preacher's kid, I dug the idea of some basic commandments. Just like the OG commandments that Moses lugged down on stone tablets, they operate as a guide for our relational interactions, without weighing near as much, thankfully.

1. Consent for sex (and any other behaviors you are asking someone to engage in) cannot be given by people who are drunk. Or under the influence of drugs. Or hardcore medications. People under the influence are already doing seriously dumb stuff, like craving those two for a dollar tacos from Jack in the Box. So don't add something to their regret list that has large, long-term consequences.

2. Going through a lot of emotional stuff can be just as bad for your decision-making process as being drunk. If someone is stressed out or dealing with a lot, they may be seeking comfort and connection, and we often equate that with sex. If you think someone isn't making a good decision, put sex on hold and be there for them in other ways—like ones that won't embarrass them a week from now.

3. Consent isn't static. Agreeing to something on one occasion does not mean agreeing to it forever. So I let you borrow my car last week. Maybe you brought it back with the gas tank empty and full of used Starbucks cups and candy wrappers and I don't want you using it again. Maybe you took fantastic care of it, but I still don't want you using it again. Either way, it's still my car, not yours. You don't just march in my house, grab the keys off the counter, and take off in my car because I let you do it last week. No consent equals Grand Theft Auto, right?

4. Consent for one thing isn't consent for another. Someone gets naked in front of you? This is an excellent sign, yes. Is it consent for any specific sexual activity? No. Agreeing to one kind of activity isn't agreeing to all of them. Making out

doesn't mean oral sex is cool. And yes to oral sex doesn't mean yes to penetrative sex. Our interactions are a salad bar, not a casserole. Wanting croutons doesn't mean you also have to have bell peppers, yanno?

5. Silence isn't consent. Someone may not actively say "no," but being passive isn't a "yes." Many times individuals don't speak up because they are freaked out or don't know how to. They could be quietly unhappy or quietly enjoying themselves. You don't know if you don't ask.

6. Consent needs to be informed. Are you sleeping with other people? That's ok, it's called dating not getting married for a reason. Have a sexually transmitted infection? That happens, too. Moving out of state in a week? That can impact future plans a bit. Potential partners need to know all of the above and any other information that may inform their decision about sexual activity. Be grown-up enough to have the awkward conversations.

7. Consent is a community obligation, not just a personal one. We need to help support each other with gray areas of consent. Speak up if you see someone in an uncomfortable situation and back up their right to say no. Friends don't let friends listen to Nickelback, and they don't let them get into situations where they are not really giving consent or not really getting consent. If you see someone at a party getting into a danger zone, then be the protective wingperson. And if the DJ plays Nickelback, it's time to leave altogether.

8. Having to convince someone is not consent. You aren't trying to win a court case by wooing a jury member. You're awesome, right? If they aren't into you enough to realize that and you have to convince them, then they don't deserve your awesomeness. If you get a "Wellllllllll, I don't knowwwwww," respond with, "That's cool, let me know if you change your mind" and then step away from the sex.

9. Consent doesn't just mean the right to say no, it also means the right to say *yes*. Shaming people because they choose to engage in sexual activity makes active, enthusiastic consent way more complicated. Affirmative consent is difficult for many people (usually women) because they think that an enthusiastic yes means they are slutty, and that they are supposed to pretend they *don't* want sex and must be "convinced." This sends mixed messages to their partners. When are we supposed to "convince" and when are we supposed to just stop? If everyone is sexually empowered, no one ever has to be "convinced."

10. Consent is more than just sex, it's about boundaries in general. You should get people's permission to touch them for any reason (e.g., "You look like you could use a hug right now, would you like one?"). Consent extends past physical boundaries, as well. You should never force your will on others. Don't share others' information, experiences, images, or things without their permission. Don't make plans on their behalf without their permission. Don't force them to share information with you or anyone else if they are uncomfortable doing so. No matter what you think is in their best interest, unless you are their legal guardian, let them make their own decisions. You do you and let them be them.

While accountability is one of those terms that has been overused and weaponized to emotionally beat the fuck out of people, it's useful in the context of consent and boundaries. Since almost none of us were raised with these kind of consent expectations, we've likely all had boundaries violated by others *and* done some boundary violating ourselves. Now, I'm not talking about clearly awful and unlawful shit like rape here. I'm talking about the more sneaky grey areas like plying someone with drinks to intentionally lower their inhibitions. Places where we could have done so much better in terms of autonomy and respecting others.

Soul searching time...any past experiences either way? Are you still in contact with the people involved? Do you have the sort of relationship where you could have a discussion about what happened and either request or give an apology? As in *"Remember that time? I was thinking about it and I really owe you a sincere apology. I can't go back in time but I can do and be better in the future."* Or *"Remember that time? I was really uncomfortable with what was going on and I don't feel like you really respected that I didn't want to do that. We can't go back in time but I can be better at expressing my boundaries so you can be clearer on respecting them."*

You noticed that I said *"do you have the sort of relationship...?"* in this paragraph, though, right? It may not be appropriate or safe to reach out. Or they may not be interested in what you have to say, and here's a new chance to respect their boundary. A friend of mine really biffed his relationship a year ago and tried to reach out and apologize to his ex...who wasn't having it. He told me *"I need to respect her wanting to be left alone. It's the least I can do, right?"*

If you think of someone you may have hurt in the past, what do you need to do to make sure it doesn't happen again in the future? It may be as simple as realizing *"I never thought about it that way. Now I know that 'convincing' someone is actually shitty and sketch and I'm over it."* Or it may mean, *"I really shouldn't drink that much, I'm far more likely to be a dick to other people when I do."* Here's a chance to make a commitment to yourself about your future interactions.

Questions for Reflection

- How were boundaries presented to you when you were younger? How has that informed the ways you treat others now and expect to be treated?
- If someone hurt you in the past, how do you need to better understand and stand your ground regarding your boundaries?
- If you hurt someone in the past, what amends can you make and how can you act differently from here on out?

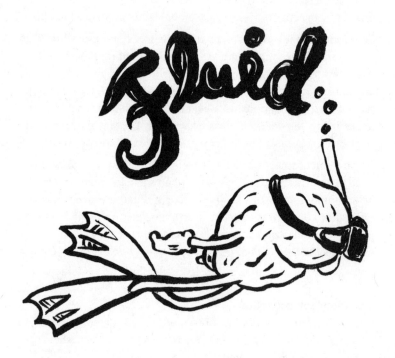

Exploring Your Sexual Identity

We have recently seen great progress in the acceptance of how truly diverse, fluid, and interesting sexual orientation is. But we have also seen continuous pushback from those who want to erase identities that they don't understand or that are not able to be neatly categorized.

Maybe you're trying to figure out your own sexual identity, or maybe you want to better understand a loved one's experience. All the competing messages out there make it difficult for many people to figure out who they really are. Since I haven't found a way to envelop everyone in a judgement-free zone bubble while they explore their sexual identity, I figure I *can* provide the best factual, evidence-based information about sexual identity I can find in order to support your process.

Sexuality Is Fluid

We're queer AF, y'all.

There was a big kerfluffle in 2016 when the trend forecasting agency J. Walter Thompson Innovation Group put out the following survey results. Only 48 percent of Gen Zs (people born from 1995 to 2010) identify as exclusively heterosexual. *Less than half.* But it's not like we suddenly queered-out in one generational shift. Their survey of millennials (ages 21 to 34 at the time of the survey) showed that only 65% considered themselves exclusively heterosexual. So not a majority, but still pretty damn queer.

Why this shift? What's causing it? Environmental toxins? Impending armageddon? The musical stylings of Miley Cyrus? Hillary Clinton's emails?

Or maybe we've just always been this way. After all, fluid sexual orientation (and gender identity) existed without rancor in many places before colonialism. Alfred Kinsey (toothbrush dude, yes) realized back in the 40s that sexuality exists on a spectrum...hence the creation of his famous Kinsey Scale. The Kinsey Scale was the attempt to rate and quantify where people fall on the spectrum of heterosexual (a zero) to homosexual (a six). Kinsey also found people who didn't fit anywhere on that scale—more on that later.

Sexuality is fluid. It's also fluid *across our lifespan*. Where you land on the Kinsey Scale today is not necessarily where you will be in a decade. Or where you were a decade ago. Per research, women are more likely to change their sexual orientation over time than men. But a lot of us have the capacity to have our head turned by someone we never expected. I'm a sex therapist with short hair who teaches yoga. It's a common assumption that my partner would be a woman. My response when people ask is, *"Nope, but the day ain't over."*

In 1948, Kinsey wrote *"The living world is a continuum in each and every one of its aspects."* Queer is just how we roll. There is literally nothing new here.

Except for the first time since the industrial revolution, we've opened the door to better exploring the experience of human attraction This means creating the language we need to support our experiences. Language informs our thoughts which informs our identity.

Many people do not need a language label (like gay, queer, straight, or pan) to validate their existence. Which I totally appreciate. But for many others, realizing that something exists, that it has a word, means that they can claim it. That they exist. And others like them exist who they can connect to. And that's powerful shit. So let's talk language.

Monosexuality means you have one category of attraction. You are either hetero or homosexual. Monosexism is widely presumed to be how all of us roll, but clearly it ain't. In fact when you look at the LGBT stats, the majority of folx are *not* monosexual.

Polysexuality is the opposite of monsexuality. It just means that you are attracted to more than one gender. This doesn't necessarily mean all genders, just more than one. It's different from early exploration or hesitation before fully coming out. And it's not just a porn trope. There are millions of people who experience sexual attraction that doesn't confine itself to a singular gender identity. There are far more polysexual people than there are gay or lesbian people.

One reason that this is all important to talk about is that individuals who are non-monosexual face greater discrimination than their gay and lesbian counterparts within the LGBT+ community in regards to medical care, mental health care, and employment. Bi women are twice as likely to be assaulted than other women and bi men also have an increased risk.

We can use polysexual as an umbrella term. It used to be that the only polysexual label was "**bisexual**" (which is why toothbrush guy's scale is now pretty outdated). There are plenty of people who find that bisexual doesn't fit their sexual orientation, and the term **pansexual** has gained more attention in the process. And, also thanks to Deadpool. Bisexuality implies a binary attraction, at least in definition, while individuals who embrace pansexuality as their identity generally express that they can experience attraction to individuals with a wide variety of gender identities, not just men or women.

Though it should not be left unsaid that plenty of people who embrace the term bi also express attraction across the gender spectrum. I've found it tends to be more a generational term than anything else. People of my generation (Xers) and older (Boomers) are more likely to use the term bisexual without necessarily differentiating it from pansexuality.

Other terms include **queer** (which is an umbrella term for people who identify outside the presumed norm), **sapiosexual** (attracted to homosapiens in many shapes and forms), or **humasexual** ("I am attracted to humans. But of course, not many." –Morrissey). I'm attracted to an intellectual type more than a physical one—should we add the term **intellectasexual** to the list? I kinda dig it.

Just because you're polysexual, doesn't mean you are open to get busy with literally everyone (though no shade thrown from me if you are!). Just like Morrissey, we all have certain types of people we gravitate toward. Sometimes we just gotta *smell right* to each other, yanno?

Orientation Is Not the Same Thing as Gender, but It Is Informed by Gender

Where does gender identity come into all this, you may ask? Here's some super-basic definitions:

Gender Identity: This is who you know yourself to be. You are assigned a sex at birth which may or may not reflect your actual gender. Whatever your gender identity, it's valid and true. You are exactly who you are supposed to be and I'm really glad you share the planet with me.

Sexual Orientation: This is who you are oriented toward, in terms of romantic and sexual attraction. It is not the same thing as sexual preference. Preference is what you like to do in bed. Orientation is who you like to do it with. Your sexual orientation is a vital part of who you are. Whatever yours is, you are not broken, you don't need correction, and I'm really glad you share the planet with me.

Gender is not sexual orientation, though your gender identity may direct the label of your sexual orientation. If for example, you are a trans woman and are attracted to men, you are a straight woman. If you had been attracted to men pre-transition, you may have been labeled (or identified) as a gay man.

If you are in a partnership with someone who is transitioning or has transitioned from the gender identity you initially understood them to have, it may or may not affect your perception of your own sexual orientation. It may feel more fluid at this point. Or it may simply be that your orientation hasn't changed, but you continue to be in love with the person you fell in love with, since their fundamental selfhood has not changed.

And if you don't have a binary gender identity (that is, neither male nor female), then how you describe your attraction alignment can get even more complicated. If you're non-binary or agender and you like women, does that make you straight or a lesbian? Neither, right? We don't have great language for these cases, so saying, "I'm genderqueer and I date women" is a mouthful but might be the most accurate.

Obviously, there is a shit-ton of additional information about gender identity that we aren't getting into here. But the important takeaway? If your identity isn't easily explained or understood by others, the reality is that you don't owe an explanation to anyone who is not living in your relationship at this moment. Fuck 'em if they don't get it.

Asexuality

Asexuality is a sexual orientation characterized by a persistent lack of sexual attraction toward any gender. –Asexuality Archive

So we got all that fluid polysexual info down. But, *hah*, we ain't done yet. Guess what? Even with all those categories, we still have a group of people who will step up and say "hell, naw" to all of them.

All the asexuals quietly minding their business, preferring chocolate cake to sex, are now thinking, "Oh, shit, she's bringing us into the equation?" Yes, my ace buddies, you deserve a place in the conversation, too. So let's tackle some ace fundamentals.

Asexuality is sort of the forgotten orientation. It's been referred to as the third orientation in a lot of literature, but of course that presumes that the other two are gay or straight.

According to a 2004 study, at least 1% of people qualify for this orientation (though the researcher notes that if you aren't interested in sex, you probably aren't interested in surveys about sex, so it might be higher). But don't forget, this isn't new data. Kinsey had a Category X in his research: About 1.5% of his respondents weren't interested in sex with *anyone*, and therefore didn't fit on his scale. So the asexual (ace) identity isn't a newfangled thing that kids these days invented on Tumblr.

Ace people are not fundamentally broken or mentally ill. It's all about our level of attraction. If there is such a huge variety of ways to feel attraction, doesn't it make sense that some people have a *none of the above* button?

If you're asexual, you might choose to never have sex. But it's not the same as celibacy or abstinence. Celibacy and abstinence are about action, not attraction. If you choose not to engage in sexual activity because of religious values, a trauma history, or other life circumstances, that's a choice you make. It's not about to whom you are attracted, but your behavior around your attraction. Asexuality, on the other hand, is about your actual level of attraction. Not everyone who is ace never has sex. You might choose to have sex because a partner desires that connection, or to conceive, or for a multitude of other reasons. But the sex itself? A means to an end, not something you are interested in for its own sake.

Being ace doesn't mean you don't experience love. Although you may be aromantic (aro), meaning that you don't experience romantic attraction any more than you experience sexual attraction. But there are plenty of ace people who are heteroromantic (experiencing romantic attraction to people of the opposite sex), homoromantic, biromantic, or panromantic. Sexual attraction and romantic attraction are two different ways of relating to other people. You can absolutely be aromantic without being asexual. And being aromantic doesn't mean you don't experience love at all, just not *romantic* love. Aro people can still experience intense love for friends, family, the world around them, and those adorable dogs that look like tiny Chewbaccas.

If you are ace and romantically inclined, dating another romantically-inclined person who is also ace might be ideal, though life rarely works that way. Being with someone who does experience sexual attraction doesn't mean the relationship is doomed, though it may mean more work and communication between you to find a middle ground that everyone is comfortable with.

A related pair of identities: **Demisexuals** and **graysexuals** fall under the ace umbrella but have a few differences. To invoke huge generalities, demisexual individuals usually only experience sexual attraction when they feel a strong emotional connection to someone. Graysexual individuals only feel sexual attraction to someone under certain circumstances, which may or may not correlate with their level of emotional intimacy.

Of the individuals I have worked with over the years, more identify as demisexual than graysexual or ace. They often seek help because they are struggling to maintain the level of sexual intimacy that their partner desires. It's something they are just not wired to have on the forefront of their minds, so we work on building the emotional attachment that helps them feel more secure and invested.

One more: Some people are not ace/gray/or demi and still love partnered sex, but their pleasure comes from pleasing a partner. The term you will generally see for this is **stone**, coming from Les Feinberg's novel *Stone Butch Blues*. And I have found that *many* different people identify as or experience their sexuality as stone.

Exploring Your Orientation

There may have been zero new words or concepts in this chapter for you. Which probably means you have already done a lot of work around understanding identity. But for a lot of folx, this may be seriously new information which means some new shit to think about it.

This is where I remind you that all of this is *fluid*. Questions arise all throughout our lifespan about our attraction to others. My youngest client currently grappling with this issue is in junior high and the oldest is in their 60s. Fluidity in orientation is a normal, healthy, good thing. And embracing who you have been, who you are now, and possibilities for the future are what help us grow as human beings.

Some questions to consider about your sexual orientation:

- What kinds of thoughts do you have regarding sexual attraction? Who do you find yourself noticing? What piques your interest? What kinds of fantasies have you had? (Fantasies don't always equate things you are actually interested in, but can sometimes provide a good clue.) What do you find erotic? What do you find yourself craving?

- To whom do you find yourself emotionally attached, and under what circumstances? What do you look for in terms of emotional closeness? In what ways have you experienced emotional attraction to someone?

- What types of sexual experiences have you had? Not just sex but also foreplay. Kissing. Even non-sexual touch that ended up being a turn on for you. What did you enjoy? What did you not enjoy?

- Have you ever experienced internal conflict regarding your attractions or lack thereof? What was the source of the conflict? What steps have you taken to address that?

- Have you ever experienced external conflict or erasure based on your attractions or lack thereof? Or been told that your identity is not valid? What steps have you taken to address that?

- What is your current relationship configuration, if any? (Example: Maybe you're pansexual but currently in a heterosexual relationship.) Have people tried to define or label you based on that relationship, therefore disregarding the complexity of who you are? What steps have you taken to address that?

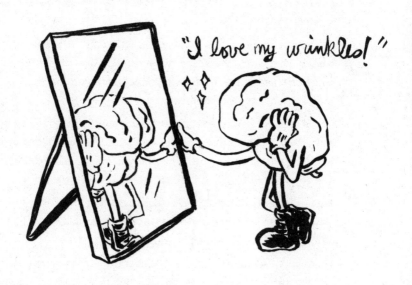

Reconnecting with Your Body

Having the words to better describe who we are can be powerful magic. But do you know what's even more bad-ass? Feeling comfortable in your skin and accepting your perfectly imperfect self.

I know how fucking difficult this is. It's a complicated, ongoing process that is often deeply uncomfortable. And that's exactly what makes it *all the more necessary to do*. This chapter is going to look at how these issues get their hooks into us, plus exercises to help us come back home to our bodies.

One major trigger for disconnecting from our physical selves is trauma. Another is just plain being unhappy with our bodies. Self-image related to physical appearance is one of the biggest barriers I have seen individuals and couples work to overcome in their quest for healthy intimacy. I've provided more context on each of these issues, and exercises designed to help in each situation (but all the exercises will help, no matter the reason for your mind-body disconnection).

Trauma, Disconnect, and Dissociation

How often are we really *in* our bodies? Rarely. And for some people, literally never.

At a fairly young age we realize that our bodies can be in one place, while our minds can wander somewhere else entirely. If third grade science was boring, our minds could already be out on the playground monkey bars. Once we learn this skill, it becomes increasingly difficult to keep our minds grounded to the present and connected to our bodies. We are always off on the proverbial monkey bars instead of being where we actually, physically are.

When we are trying to increase our intimacy with another person, reconnecting our minds and bodies to be present can be intensely difficult. To say it as simply as I do to my clients on the regular, your partner (hopefully) wants to have sex *with* you, not *on* you. This means you have to be engaged, not just to their experience and pleasure, but to your own.

Interoception is the fancy clinical term used to describe our awareness of our body's reactions. If perception is how we know what is going on around us, interoception is how we know what is going on *inside* us.

This is often a super foreign concept, especially for people with trauma histories. Dissociation from our experiences is a form of protection in fucked-up situations. If someone is harming us and we can't escape physically, we escape mentally. But getting back into our bodies when we are safe to do so can seem impossible. Research demonstrates that people with severe trauma histories often have significant differences in the areas of their brain mapped as interoceptive pathways.

A lot of us without trauma histories still struggle with interoception. Trauma reactions aren't the only cause of body disconnect. Body image bullshit is nearly universal. All kinds of shame issues can trigger disassociation. And that means we aren't connected to how our body is reacting, so we are not connected to how it is affecting our emotions, and   do not have a conscious awareness of our behaviors. When we don't practice interoception, we struggle to act with purpose. Including in regard to healthy sexual intimacy.

Interoception Exercise

This exercise is designed to build interoception. It's adapted from Peter Levine's fantastic book *In An Unspoken Voice*:

Hold out one of your hands. It doesn't matter which one, but take note of your choice. Hold it in the air, without letting it rest against another surface (like a table top or your leg).

Open up the palm of that hand, facing back toward your body, and use your eyes to observe it.

Slowly make a fist with that hand, watching the whole time. Take note when your hand feels completely closed into a fist.

Without breaking eye contact, open your hand back up.

Now close your eyes, and repeat this exercise.

Feel what open feels like from the inside, then the act of closing your hand into a fist, then reopening. Pay attention to all that you notice in your body that wasn't present when you were focusing on your external sight messages.

How did your awareness of the experience change once you were entirely dependent on your internal sensory messages? Was it disconcerting at any point? Comforting? Did anything shift or feel different in how you connected with yourself?

Progressive Muscle Relaxation

The purpose of this exercise is to gain awareness of how our body is operating from the inside. You know, that interoception thing I was yammering on about. Actively engaging in progressive muscle relaxation effectively loosens and relaxes the muscles. By tightening a muscle and then releasing it, you can feel the difference between tense and relaxed.

Make sure not to do any movements that cause pain. If any of these exercises cause discomfort, ease up or stop. Sometimes if you are very tense already, actively tensing your muscles with a progressive muscle relaxation exercise will not be helpful. If this is the case, you may want to try passive progressive muscle relaxation exercises instead (focus on relaxing parts of your body, rather than tensing and then relaxing to feel the difference).

Here is a script for the guided progressive muscle relaxation exercise. You can read it as you go or have someone read it to you:

Find a comfortable position sitting, standing, or lying down. You can change positions at any time during the exercise.

Breathe in forcefully and deeply, and hold this breath. Hold it... hold it... and now release. Let all the air go out slowly, and release all the tension.

Take another deep breath in. Hold it... and then exhale slowly, allowing the tension to leave your body with the air.

Now breathe even more slowly and gently... breathe in... hold... out... breathe in... hold... out...

Continue to breathe slowly and gently. Allow your breathing to relax you.

Focus on the large muscles of your legs. Tighten all your leg muscles. Now tense them even further. Hold onto this tension. Feel how tight and tense the muscles in your legs are right now. Squeeze the muscles harder, tighter... Continue to hold this tension. Feel the muscles wanting to give up this tension. Hold it for a few moments more... and now relax. Let all the tension go. Feel the muscles in your legs going limp, loose, and relaxed. Notice how relaxed the muscles feel now. Feel the difference between tension and relaxation. Enjoy the pleasant feeling of relaxation in your legs.

Now focus on the muscles in your arms. Tighten your shoulders, upper arms, lower arms, and hands. Squeeze your hands into tight fists. Tense the muscles in your arms and hands as tightly as you can. Squeeze harder... harder... hold the tension in your arms, shoulders, and hands. Feel the tension in these muscles. Hold it for a few moments more... and now release. Let the muscles of your shoulders, arms, and hands relax and go limp. Feel the relaxation as your shoulders lower into a comfortable position and your hands relax at your sides. Allow the muscles in your arms to relax completely.

Focus again on your breathing. Slow, even, regular breaths. Breathe in relaxation...and breathe out tension...in relaxation...and out tension... Continue to breathe slowly and rhythmically.

Now focus on the muscles of your buttocks. Tighten these muscles as much as you can. Hold this tension... and then release. Relax your muscles.

Tighten the muscles of your back now. Feel your back tightening, pulling your shoulders back and tensing the muscles along your spine.

Arch your back slightly as you tighten these muscles. Hold... and relax. Let all the tension go. Feel your back comfortably relaxing into a good and healthy posture.

Turn your attention now to the muscles of your chest and stomach. Tighten and tense these muscles. Tighten them further... hold this tension... and release. Relax the muscles of your trunk.

Finally, tighten the muscles of your face. Scrunch your eyes shut tightly, wrinkle your nose, and tighten your cheeks and chin. Hold this tension in your face... and relax. Release all the tension. Feel how relaxed your face is.

Notice all of the muscles in your body... notice how relaxed your muscles feel. Allow any last bits of tension to drain away. Enjoy the relaxation you are experiencing. Notice your calm breathing... your relaxed muscles... Enjoy the relaxation for a few moments...

When you are ready to return to your usual level of alertness and awareness, slowly begin to re-awaken your body. Wiggle your toes and fingers. Swing your arms gently. Shrug your shoulders. Stretch if you like.

You may now end this progressive muscle relaxation exercise feeling calm and refreshed.

Body Image

Body image issues can arise for a billion different reasons. All of us eventually experience some kind of unwanted body changes due to accident, injury, giving birth, or just getting older. Other people struggle with their overall size, height, hair or lack of it, or how certain parts of their bodies stack up to traditional beauty standards.

Folx with gender dysphoria may struggle greatly with a body that has features out of alignment with their true gender. Most everyone struggles with some aspect of the skin suit they wear around during their time on the planet.

Anxious and negative thoughts about our bodies are so commonplace they have become the new normal. Fun fact: approximately 80% of women report feeling dissatisfied with their bodies. A *Glamour* study found that the average woman says 13 negative statements about her body to herself on a given day (one per hour of being awake, on average). 97% had *at least* one negative statement in a day.

But body image issues are no longer primarily the domain of women, if they ever were. A UK study looking body image among women and men and found that 75% of women and almost 81% of men experience anxiety related to their body. The number of men struggling with body image is starting to match, and in some places, surpass that of women. No one is safe from the self-destruction we impose on ourselves with negative body image self-talk. Male body issues are something we talk about quite rarely. In trying to do something about that, my friend Aaron Sapp and I wrote a zine specifically about male body image issues. It's called *Detox Your Masculinity*, if you are looking for more resources and ideas.

So how do you unfuck your body image? Studies of individuals who have positive images of their body show an interesting trend. The majority of people with a positive image of their physical self had actively done work to combat a negative body image at some point in their lives. They had developed an awareness of the issue and worked on changing it in a conscious way, rather than hitting the gym, going on the latest on-trend diet, or investing in tons of plastic surgery. Doing things to feel healthy and good about yourself is awesome, but if you don't do the *inside* work the outside work doesn't truly fix anything.

As is true about most research, these studies didn't look at the lived experience of non-cis people, so I can only speak from my practice as a therapist in this regard. Gender dysphoria (for those who experience it… and you can absolutely have a non-cis identity without experiencing dysphoria) is a very real struggle that I would never discount by saying *"let's work on a more positive body image!"*

I have found it most helpful to partner with my non-cis clients on how to care for the body they have now, so they are the healthiest they can be when they do receive gender congruence treatments (e.g., managing hormone side effects, preparing for surgeries). The focus of the internal work is on validating their authentic identity, not just finding peace with the body they currently have. I've used the phrase *"Despite others' perceptions or opinions about me, I know who I am"* as a hypnotherapy affirmation. It's a small shift in thinking that has given many people the support they truly needed.

The exercises in this chapter are designed to help with the inside work, both as an individual and with a romantic partner. If you do not have active body issues (and if so, congratulations you rare gem, you!) you may still benefit from these exercises. Connecting to your body through awareness exercises can promote increased intimacy, even for people who are already generally body-confident.

You can complete these exercises by yourself or with a partner. It can be helpful, in partnered relationships, to have the person who is most comfortable with their body complete and share the exercises first. This can create a safe zone for the less comfortable partner to do the same. Or if you're anxious about sharing, it might be more helpful for you to try the exercises on your own first. If you are doing these exercises by yourself, you can then consider which aspects of the experience you are willing to share with a current or future partner.

Also, keep in mind that there are trained body workers (in all their shapes and forms) available in many communities to help guide you through these exercises, which can be helpful for people who struggle with following along in a workbook and who can benefit from a more direct teaching experience. Check out the Institute for Mind Body Therapy as a good starting point to find a body worker who matches with your particular needs. Body work can encompass a lot of different things, including surrogate partner therapy, massage therapy, therapeutic touch work, somatic experiencing, and a host of other interventions that involve working with a hands-on practitioner.

The goals of these exercises are:

- To feel more connected to and comfortable with your physical body

- To feel more connected and comfortable with your partner's physical body

- To gain empathy for your partner's body image issues, if present

- To identify any body image issues you may be experiencing

- To build respect and appreciation for the strength and functionality of your body

- To cultivate persistent, gentle curiosity about the experience of being human

Clothed Body Work

This is another activity designed to help you build your interoception and enhance your comfort and acceptance of your external, physical self.

If you are working with a partner during this activity, discuss in advance their role in the process. The important thing is that they listen to your words rather than correct anything you say, especially your thoughts and feelings. We often want to tell our partners how we perceive them, and we often see them with much less criticism than they see themselves. It's hard not to say something akin to "No! I love your neck!" The point of the exercise is to share our own internal experience without fear of argument or correction.

It is also not your partner's job to ask questions or give feedback about your experience. The partner's job is to provide a supportive presence, then complete the activity with your support as well. It's amazing what you will learn about each other, if you are in a place where you feel safe enough to do this activity together.

Stand in front of a full-length mirror, wearing whatever clothing feels comfortable (as much or as little as you'd like). Take a deep breath and look at your body in its entirety for a few minutes. If this isn't something you often do, give yourself time to become accustomed to the experience.

Starting at the top of your head and moving downward, describe out loud each part of your body and the feelings you have about each part. If you are doing this activity alone, still say everything you are thinking out loud. It is amazing how much we say to ourselves that we are not aware of, because we don't give literal voice to those thoughts and feelings. When you're done, ask yourself some of these questions:

- What did you notice about yourself? Did anything surprise you? Did anything you found yourself saying out loud surprise you?

- If you were to pick out one or two body parts/areas that you most dislike, what would these be and why? You can be present for these feelings, acknowledge them, and work to generate self-compassion for your experience.

- If you were to pick out one or two body parts/areas that are your favorite, what would they be and why?

- Did your perceptions of yourself shift when you moved from looking at your entire body to focusing on parts of it at a time? If so, in what ways?

- If you did this activity with a partner, please ask your partner to answer the following questions: What surprised you about your partner's experience? Did they say anything you didn't expect? Did you notice that they ignored any areas? Express any thoughts or feelings that you weren't aware of?

Nude Body Work

Now, you are going to complete the same exercise, but without clothing.

If you are doing this exercise with a partner, undress, acknowledge the expected nervousness, and give permission to look at one another's bodies. Hold hands and look together for a couple of minutes, then take turns looking at each other's backside.

If becoming completely nude immediately, whether alone or with a partner, makes you uncomfortable, you can disrobe slowly as you complete the exercise. You can also incorporate softer lighting and soothing music if you find that helpful, but you don't want ambient music to be a distraction or have lighting so low you can't really see yourself.

Repeat the above steps, speaking all your thoughts and feelings about each part of yourself out loud (or writing them down if that feels more comfortable...I know this already feels weird!), and consider these questions:

- What did you notice about yourself? Did anything surprise you? Did anything you found yourself saying out loud that surprised you? Was there anything different from the clothed version of this exercise?

- If you were to pick out one or two body parts/areas that you most dislike, what would these be and why? Was there anything different from the clothed version of this exercise?

- If you were to pick out one or two body parts/areas that are your favorite, what would they be and why? Was there anything different from the clothed version of this exercise?

- Did your perceptions of yourself shift when you moved from looking at your entire body to focusing on parts of it at a time? If so, in what ways? Was there anything different from the clothed version of this exercise?

- If you did this activity with a partner, please ask your partner to answer the following questions. What surprised you about your partner's experience? Did they say anything you didn't expect? Express any thoughts or feelings that you weren't aware of? Did you notice that they skipped over any areas? Did anything different happen from the clothed version of this exercise?

Some Tips for Being More Accepting of Your Own Body

- Focus on an aspect of yourself that is separate from the destructive body image messages you are combating. Consider this aspect a different dimension from what you are unhappy about. Focus on your strong self, playful self, sensual self, etc. and let that aspect become engaged during sexual intimacy.

- Focus on your body in its entirety, rather than certain parts. Look at yourself and ask your partner to look at you with "soft eyes," or focusing on the entirety of what you, and they, love, appreciate, and respect about you. This may be easier to believe than *"I love your eyes"* and *"I think your butt is sexy."*

- Hold space for the possibility that even if you do not accept and love your body right now, it is possible to feel differently in the future. *"Not right now"* has far less a pervasive hold on us than *"never,"* and allows small shifts to occur that move us in a healthy direction.

- When positivity seems completely impossible, work toward neutrality. Just like "not right now," neutrality is far less damaging self-talk than continued negativity. When you catch yourself saying something negative to yourself and a positive statement seems like unbearable bullshit when you feel awful, try something along the lines of *"My body just is. Nothing is empirically good or bad. My body and I are doing the best we can."*

- Apologize (as authentically as possible, even if it feels cheesy) to your body for treating it like the enemy. For treating it like it is somehow a separate entity from the rest of you. Tell it you will work on incorporating it back into the whole and appreciate all it has done to keep you moving forward despite your negativity toward it.

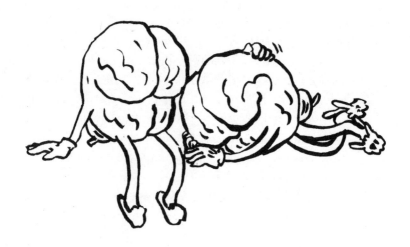

Your Sense of Touch

I have perceiv'd that to be with those I like is enough,
To stop in company with the rest at evening is enough,
To be surrounded by beautiful, curious, breathing, laughing flesh is enough,
To pass among them or touch any one, or rest my arm ever so lightly round
his or her neck for a moment, what is this then?
I do not ask any more delight, I swim in it as in a sea.

There is something in staying close to men and women and looking on
them, and in the contact and odor of them, that pleases the soul well,
All things please the soul, but these please the soul well.
        —Walt Whitman, from "I Sing The Body Electric" in *Leaves of Grass*

A friend told me recently that he knew his marriage was over when his wife wouldn't let him touch her anymore. He was by no means the first person to tell me that, and unfortunately won't be the last.

The sense of touch is, when you think about it, an exercise in paradox.

Jennifer Kennerk, a Waldorf school educator, wrote how our sense of touch is the way we first learn to differentiate ourselves from the rest of the world. If we touch someone or something, we develop awareness of where we end and the other person or object begins. She states that touch "allows us to understand our own individual place in the world, and also to understand that others have their own individuality as well. The sense of touch provides human beings with the ability to understand their own uniqueness and therefore the uniqueness of others." Touch is the sense that demonstrates the boundaries between our individual bodies and the rest of the universe.

The paradox arises because touch is also our primary means of experiencing intimacy with others. Human beings are hardwired to connect, and the primary mechanism for doing so is through touch. We express closeness through touch. We experience others, gain awareness of their presence, and invite them into our own.

We also need touch to survive. In the thirteenth century, King Frederick II of Germany wanted to study language acquisition. He was curious as to whether children are born with knowledge of language or if it is something they learn from caregivers over time. He's alleged to have set up an experiment to determine if children would speak, spontaneously, if they never heard language to begin with. He took 50 babies within his kingdom and assigned them each to foster mothers. The babies had their basic needs met. They were bathed and nursed, but were not held or cuddled or talked to. *The experiment failed because all fifty infants died.*

In more recent years, the world has learned about the horrific overcrowding and miserable conditions in many orphanages in the world. Harvard Medical School researcher Mary Carlson observed the conditions in a Romanian orphanage, where due to understaffing and overcrowding, babies lay neglected in their cribs and were rarely touched, even during meal times. She observed no engagement, no crying, no babbling, and no whimpering. While their physical needs were being met, in theory, Carlson found that by age two the babies had unusually high amounts of cortisol, a stress hormone known to cause brain damage. Growth was stunted; the children acted half their age.

What conclusions can be drawn from King Frederick's failed experiment and the Romanian orphanage scandal? Lack of touch impedes the human ability to thrive. In some cases it leads to death. Caring for basic physical needs is not enough; we need touch to survive.

Those of us who did not get a lot of touching before age twelve often struggle with touch as adults. Snuggling, cuddling, hugging, and holding hands often makes us uncomfortable. And we thereby lose opportunities for connection. We communicate best through touch, as many of our ancestors did throughout the ages. Touch is universal. Touch, both sexual and non-sexual, is essential for intimacy. Non-sexual touch is an essential building block for physical intimacy.

Touch makes us more relationally honest. Studies of compliance in field settings have shown amazing results when touch was involved. In one study, researchers put a dime in the change box of a public telephone. (This study was clearly conducted in the 70s.) Study participants would go into the phone booth, make a call, and then would put their hand in the little coin receiver to see if there was any extra change. As they exited the booth, they were approached and asked, *"Did you find any money in the change box in the telephone booth?"* 97% lied and said no. But in the same experiment, if the researcher reached out and touched the individual on the shoulder while asking the question, 95% told the truth. They would say they found money there and would offer it to the person who asked.

The famous family therapist Virginia Satir said that we need four hugs a day for survival, eight for maintenance, and twelve for growth.

Do you get the amount of touch that you need in a day? Depending on the country you live in, maybe not.

Psychologist Sidney Journal studied touch by observing couples dining in various countries and counted the number of times they touched each other. On average, in Mexico City, couples touched each other 185 times an hour; in Paris it was 115 times an hour. In

London, couples did not touch each other at all and in Gainesville, Florida it was twice an hour.

The couples in Mexico City did not engage in passionate kisses 185 times an hour (no time to eat their dinner!) but they stroked each other's arms, or hair. Leaned into each other. Continued to convey the message that they desired each other. They communicated their connection to each other through different levels of touch.

Understanding What Touch Means to You

The idea that there are different levels of touch is wild to many people. It definitely isn't something that we talk about. The concept of five levels of touch comes from the work of clinical sexologist Dr. Patti Britton, whose work has informed mine for many years now.

Go through these questions and write down your answers. If you are partnered, consider having your partner answer these questions separately from you, then compare your answers:

- The first level of touch is healing. What does that mean to you? What kind of touch do you consider healing? What kind of healing touch do you enjoy receiving? Giving?

- The second level of touch is affectionate. What does that mean to you? What kind of touch do you consider affectionate? What kind of affectionate touch do you enjoy receiving? Giving?

- The third level of touch is sensual. What does that mean to you? What kind of touch do you consider sensual? What kind of sensual touch do you enjoy receiving? Giving?

- The fourth level of touch is erotic. What does that mean to you? What kind of touch do you consider erotic? What kind of erotic touch do you enjoy receiving? Giving?

- The fifth level of touch is sexual. What does that mean to you? What kind of touch to you consider sexual? What kind of sexual touch do you enjoy receiving? Giving?

I've had many people complete this exercise over the years and come back and tell me that it really blew their minds. That, for example, they hadn't considered a difference between sensual and erotic touch, and realized that sensual touch was something they really were missing and craved.

The process is as deeply individual and unique as everything else that we do as people. There is no right or wrong, there are just *your* definitions. If you do this exercise with a partner and they have wildly different definitions, that's OK, too. You are discovering some really important shit about yourself and them. The point isn't to fit into a box, it's to understand our own experiences and how those impact our connections with others.

More Questions to Consider

- Of the kinds of touch you described above, which do you enjoy most? What makes you feel safe? Desired?

- What kind of touch makes you feel uncomfortable?

- Does your interest in touch, or the different types of touch you typically enjoy, change when you are feeling strong (possibly negative) emotions? How so? Are you aware of these changes at the time or is it something you notice in retrospect?

- If you are partnered, in your experience, what kind of touch does your partner(s) most respond to?

- Have you and your partner(s) experienced any issues or struggles with touch in your relationship(s)? How so?

- If a partner also did some reflecting on the levels of touch, did any of their answers surprise you? What surprised you most? How do you think that knowing different information about them may change your relationship?

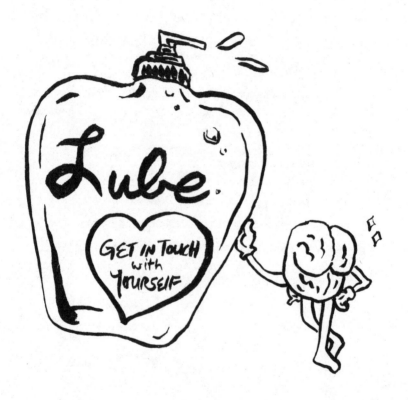

Sexing Yourself

"Everyone does it, but no one admits it."

This statement almost always refers to one of two human activities. One is eating Jack in the Box egg rolls at 3 a.m. The other is masturbation.

Masturbation is simply the touching of one's genitals for the purpose of sexual pleasure and is part of the normal human expression of sexuality. It is a healthy and empowering practice that leads to better sex lives, and it's just something people do. Like brushing our teeth, baking cookies, or playing board games, it's a normal human behavior.

Historical records and anthropological studies indicate that masturbation has always been a part of human history. In the grand tradition of ruining anything fun, the public tides turned against the art of self-love as society "modernized" and an organized movement against the practice of masturbation began. Religious leaders and medical professionals became outspoken regarding their views that masturbation was dangerous. It led to weakness, disease, and insanity, they said. It was decried as an affront to God.

Only in the past 50 years have researchers like Alfred Kinsey (hey there, toothbrush dude!), William Masters, Virginia Johnson, and Betty Dodson begun confronting these views of masturbation. They all argued that masturbation is a healthy, normal, and valuable part of human development. Dodson specifically encouraged women to masturbate as an act of feminist resistance to negative images of womanhood common in many families, religious organizations, and society in general. Dodson also proposed using masturbation as a way of enhancing self-esteem, and perhaps most importantly, as the best means of becoming orgasmic.

Despite their work, there remains a prevailing attitude about the inherent wrongness of masturbation that we can't seem to shake.

Sigh.

So let me add my voice to the mix.

Masturbation is not a sin. It is not a shameful practice. It is way healthier than fast food at 3 a.m., and it shouldn't be so damn secretive. As Betty Dodson states in her book *Sex for One: The Joy of Selfloving*: "Our cultural denial of masturbation sustains sexual repression." How else are you going to know what you like and then communicate that to present or future partners?

I am raising kids who are open and self-confident. The work that I do is embarrassing enough for them, so I won't detail the conversations we have in our home—but I have always normalized masturbation as a way of relieving stress and maintaining control of their sexual selves. If and when they choose partnered sexual activity, it will be an educated and empowered choice made with as much information available to them as possible.

And masturbation is just as important for us grown people. Whether you're single or partnered, enjoying sexual release through masturbation can be both relaxing and liberating.

I've been asked, *Doesn't this make me a total loser?* This question somehow implies that masturbation is an inferior form of sex, and what the fuck is up with that? In the age of Craigslist, anyone can find partnered sex; it isn't like you somehow win extra points because someone was willing to fuck you silly. This question also presumes that if you are masturbating, then you *don't* have someone around who is fucking you silly, which isn't always the case.

Not all sex has to be partnered, and scrounging up a partner-person may not be on your agenda for the afternoon. Why should it be? Taking care of yourself and having a nice orgasm doesn't have to *always* be a team effort.

When working with single individuals who want to prevent future relationship mistakes, I encourage them to get in touch with their body and find out what they like and don't like. This may include exercise, massage, touch exercises (like the ones in this book!), and/or masturbation. You are far less likely to rush into a poor partner choice if you know what you want in a relationship before you start looking.

For those of us who are already partnered? Just because we are already having sex with someone else doesn't mean we can't also have sex with ourselves—whether to relax, learn more about ourselves, or just because we want to.

No matter what age you are, and no matter what your relationship status is, if you aren't sure what turns you on, isn't it time to start finding out?

Why Is Masturbation Important?

Sexual expression should be an empowering part of your experience as a human being. We live in a world that is continuously disempowering, and we get all kinds of competing and fucked-up messages about what it means to be a sexual being. The reality is, there are as many answers as there are people on the planet.

Exploring your sexuality with a partner is a wonderful thing, should you have or want to have a partner at the time. But sex with someone else is as much about them and the connection you create by being together as it is about figuring out your own body. Solo sex is *just for you* and can have an entirely different intent. Such as:

- Figuring out what you like—for yourself, or to share with future partners if you are so inclined to have them

- Reclaiming your sexuality from the fucked-up shit you've dealt with in your past

- Reclaiming your sexuality from the fucked-up messages our culture inundate us with on a constant basis

- Healing from trauma

- Empowering yourself, Betty Dodson style

- Political activism to actively fight sexual repression

- You've got a headache. Or cramps

- You are having trouble falling asleep

- Because orgasms feel good, duh!

- Because WHYTHEFUCKNOT?

What Do I *Do*, Though?

Turn yourself on: figure out where and how you like to be touched and touch away.

There are lots of places on the human body that are erogenous, meaning they connect you to your sexual self. When erogenous areas are stimulated, you find yourself sexually aroused. So, start touching. Your breasts and nipples and all aspects of your genitalia, your perineum, your anus, your G-spot. Anywhere else you might like to be touched…the crease of your left pinky toe, if that does it for ya. Yes, it makes sense to stroke your clitoris if you have one, or your penis if you have one of those (and just so you know, most of the nerve endings in the penis are under the head of it).

The point is to listen to your body while you explore.

Do you like firm touch, light touch, vibrating touch, warm water from the bath faucet? If you discover touch you enjoy, blood will rush to that area (which leads to swollen erectile tissue in the clitoris, penis, or nipples). Lubricants (dry like talc powder or wet like lube or lotion) may help your sensory experience, as can sex toys in general (more on that in a minute).

The Orgasm

Rebecca Chalker writes about this in her book *The Clitoral Truth*: When we are turned on, sensory messages are sent to the brain and the brain says "woohoo!" and starts increasing the number of nerves in the body that are activated. Once one system is on high alert, it boops the next system in the chain and gets *it* going. After the whole system is activated, we reach overload. And that energy has to discharge somehow, right?

This whole chain reaction thing works best with certain rhythmic cycles, which are very much linked to our own heartbeats. This is our "excitability cycle." We all have our own rhythm. Which makes sense, because not everyone has the exact same heartbeat cadence, right? You know your own rhythm best, or want to find out. So, explore.

Masturbation lets you figure out your own dance steps without having to dance in sync with someone else. And yay for that.

I realize that not everyone is naturally orgasmic. You may be reading this right now out of frustration about, or fear of, that being true for you. There are a lot of things that can affect our ability to be orgasmic, generally falling under one of the following categories:

- **Physical Issues.** For example, medical things you have going on or medications you are taking. If you are struggling in that regard, going to a doctor to see if there's a physical cause makes a lot of sense. And it may be an easy fix. For example, if your antidepressant is decreasing your sex drive, your doc can switch it up or add something to mitigate that side effect.

- **Emotional Issues**. For example, if you have had sexual trauma, that can play a huge role in shutting down your sexual responses. But it doesn't have to be something so big and complicated as that. Some people got so many negative messages about sex growing up that they have become insidious mental blocks to feeling comfortable with being orgasmic. I do a lot of work with people in my private practice on unpacking some of those messages and reclaiming their sexual selves.

And hey, there's good information earlier in this book about both physical and emotional issues and tips on working with those issues. And it is all information that is meant to help with both solo and partnered sex!

The larger point here is that you may be exploring yourself and not getting anywhere. And it's okay to get more help from a professional (doesn't *that* sound dirty?) to figure out if there are other things going on.

And make sure you read my chapter later on sex toys—ahem—*sexual aids*. It has lots of good info about using aids for solo sex as well as partnered sex.

What About Us Ace, Grey, Demi, and Stone People?

About 1% (ish) of the world is asexual (or demisexual, graysexual, etc.), which I talked about earlier in this book. Some of y'all have zero interest in orgasms at all. And some of y'all do have interest, just not at the same level. Or not every time a stiff wind blows past your junk.

If orgasms through masturbation are part of your life, that's great. If not, that's great, too. I just don't want anyone thinking they shouldn't masturbate because it somehow makes them a bad person. I have no more patience for shitty societal messages.

Don't masturbate if that's not your thing. But if it is your thing, and other people are telling you it shouldn't be? Who gives a fuck what they think. Get to it.

And for stone folx—people who enjoy their partner's pleasure rather than their own—it's entirely okay to not have interest in solo sex, and still want partnered sex where your sexual satisfaction comes from satisfying your partner.

What About Us Non-Cis People?

A lot of the above stuff totally may apply to you, but it also isn't fair to go, "Here is info for cisfolk. Everyone else? Your mileage may vary." So whether you are trans, nonbinary, agender, bigender, genderqueer, gender nonconforming, or *anything other than cisgender*, here is some basic information and research that is specific to gender confirmation treatments and the changes that may occur if someone is undergoing these treatments. I mean, I *am* the science-y, research-y chick and I haven't yet seen any research published around this topic and that makes me grumpy. Because gender confirmation treatments don't mean we have to give up the experience of our sexual selves, right?

Generally speaking, if you are no-hormone and/or no-op, the info for cis people applies, except for the (sometimes huge) added issue of possible dysphoria triggers. And just like any person for any reason having triggers around any kind of sex, the important thing is to find ways to work with that issue. Or around it, if need be.

For instance, you can try sensate focus work (like the exercises in Part Three) that omits areas that trigger dysphoria. Or you can find other ways to create comfort in the experience, such as leaving your binder on during sexual activity (yes, even during solo sex!). You know your body and your comfort level best, and get to set the boundaries around that experience. *Especially* in solo sex, when your focus is pleasure, exploration, and comfort.

Solo Sex After Starting Feminizing Hormone Therapy

A lot of trans women and transfem* individuals on hormone therapy (HT) who have not had a vaginoplasty note a difference in their sex drive and inclination to masturbate and/or have sex. Notice I said difference? Difference isn't bad or good…it's just not the same as before.

You may notice that your ejaculate seems more like pre-cum than a traditional load (but don't consider that me saying you can't get a fertile partner with a uterus pregnant, okay??), and a lot of folx report that it takes far more intellectual and/or emotional stimulation than it did in the past. If physical stimulation isn't enough, consider adding some of these elements before giving up.

There are also some activities you may not have even thought of engaging in before that might be something you want to try. Some no-op trans women and transfem* folx like stimulating the inguinal canals during solo (or partnered) sex as an alternative to penis stimulation. This is better known as *muffing,* and Mira Bellwether's guide to doing so can be found online if you're intrigued.

Solo Sex After Vaginoplasties

Vaginal care after a vaginoplasty is already going to be something you hear about ad nauseum, which is a good thing because it's really important. Some of the stuff you will hear about is the importance of using lubricant and using a vasaldilator for a year or so after surgery to keep your vagina from contracting closed or scarring shut. Solo sex may be a place where you incorporate post-op care for your new vulva and vagina, because you can do so in the context of enjoying yourself as a sexual being.

The best research roundup I have found for individuals who have had vaginoplasties with clitoroplasties was transresearch.info (a great resource if you haven't seen it already). The studies they cite showed that 30% of trans women had difficulty masturbating to orgasm after surgery (but it *was* doable!) and another 18% couldn't orgasm at all. Interestingly, that number decreased to 14% when all sexual activity was included, not just masturbation. This means, again, that intellectual and emotional stimulation plays a big role in our sexual satisfaction, right?

Orgasms just may take more creativity to accomplish. We've all have learned to do complicated things that have become simple with practice, and it's important to use that same mindset when focusing on our sexual pleasure. Surgically speaking, the clitoris is formed from the most sensitive area of the penis, so a clitoral orgasm is entirely possible. *But* it isn't the only way for a post-op transwoman, transfem* individual (or anyone born with a clitoris for that matter) to have an orgasm. G spot stimulation and anal stimulation thrown into the mix might be really helpful.

Solo Sex After Starting Masculinizing Hormone Treatment

So first off: if you are taking testosterone (T), congrats. If your clitoris doesn't cause dysphoria for you, you are going to reap some fun benefits. The clitoris has twice the nerve endings as the penis (8000 versus 4000), and your clitoris grows due to the T (probably around an inch or two, although there are reports of up to 3 inches), which means more of it will protrude from the hood, meaning more of those nerve endings are exposed. Which means your orgasms will likely be more intense and happen faster.

More good news: there are sexual aids designed specifically for transmen and transmasc folx who take T. Activist and porn star Buck Angel has been involved in the creation of the Buck Off (a stroker toy) and T-Lube (a lubricant specifically formulated for the dryness that can occur as a side effect of testosterone therapy).

Solo Sex After Metoidioplasty

Some transmen and transmasc folx opt for a metoidioplasty, which essentially works with the clitoris you already have (and have enlarged somewhat on T). Metoidioplasty takes the clitoris that has already been enlarged from testosterone therapy and repositions it to give additional length and place it in the usual position for a penis. This means your penis will be bioconstructed with your existing erectile tissue. While there may not be enough erectile tissue for you to penetrate a partner without a sexual aid (and I haven't seen any extenders or hollow-core strap ons designed to work specifically for someone with a metoidioplasty...we need an engineer to get on that, STAT!), you can definitely still enjoy solo sex quite easily and a sexual aid like the Buck Off will still work great.

Solo Sex After Phalloplasty

With a phalloplasty, skin grafts are collected from other places on your body to bio-construct a larger penis. But since erectile tissue can't be constructed, a penile implant will need to be used (just like it would with a cisgender man who has incurable erectile dysfunction). Less erectile tissue is salvaged with this procedure, which can decrease ability to orgasm.

But even with the phalloplasty, most transmen and transmasc folx report having more sex (of all kinds) and more sexual satisfaction. Enjoying and exploring your new penis can be empowering and enjoyable, even if you don't climax. It's another aspect of being authentically who you are, and that's awesome.

My Partner Wants to Watch, the Perv-o. What's Up with That?

Maybe they think it's hot. We are visual creatures after all. Or maybe they want to see how you touch yourself so they can better know how to touch you in the ways you like (which makes for an excellent partner).

It can feel really intimidating and vulnerable, but it can also really enhance partner intimacy. Don't rule it out. Consider how to up your comfort level by changing lighting, maybe staying partially clothed, or having them engage in masturbation at the same time as you.

Sex Toys

Sex toys, aka sexual aids, provide stimulation and sensation: vibration, movement, warmth, etc. All the stuff we create for each other and ourselves for the purpose of sexual pleasure. I wrote a zine all about sexual aids, how to shop for them, how to take care of them, and all that needful etcetera that you don't generally see.

By far the biggest question I get from people is about whether sex toys will "break" them for other types of sex, therefore ruining their sex lives. Sex toys can provide a more intensive version of sexual sensations. But that isn't gonna break anything.

Think of it this way: you can walk to the store or drive, right? If you walk it might take you awhile longer, but you're still gonna get there. Walking has its benefits. You slow down, you connect to the world around you, you enjoy the view. Walking can be a ton of fun. But sometimes you just need to run into the grocery store and grab a bag of chips before the party, you know? Nothing wrong with driving, is there?

So the other question you may have is, *"What if walking isn't getting me there and I can only get the chips from the store if I drive?"* That totally does not make you broken. It just means you need more stimulation than other people. The toy didn't create that, that's just how you're wired down there.

If that kind of bums you out, the question I would ask is: what exactly does the driving do for you that the walking doesn't? For example, if you are a clitoris-having person, you may have a clitoral hood that blocks a lot of sensation. A toy might provide the extra sensation you need to get the job done. You might be able to get a similar effect if you or your partner push back your clitoral hood during sex. Some people also have that hood pierced, so the piercing provides the stimulation. Some people have a clitoral hood reduction surgery if it's really getting in the way.

So a toy may be solving a problem you didn't really know existed until you investigate a bit further.

So many people born with penises have had circumcisions (or at least gotten decent information about pushing back their foreskin for stimulation) so that muffling of sensation is less an issue. But missing out on sensation can happen in other ways, too. Maybe your g-spot (which are not limited to vagina-having people, BTW!) is getting stimulated in just the right way by a certain toy, and that can be replicated with your or your partner's fingers. Or maybe it's your perineum (taint, durf, gooch, etc....and yes, the perineum is not limited to penis-having people) that is getting hit the right way.

Pay attention to what the toy is actually doing for you, not just the final outcome. Erm, bag of chips. Whatever.

Toys can be lifesavers for both solo and partnered sex. They are nothing to be ashamed about. Some people have mobility issues that would make masturbation impossible without them. Sometimes toys allow people to participate in sex in a way they couldn't otherwise. Individuals who struggle to maintain an erection might find using a hollow core strap helpful in still allowing them penetrative intercourse with their partner. Or someone who doesn't have a penis but wants to penetrate a partner may use a traditional strap-on. In short? Sex toys are meant to enhance our experience, not replace partners. And technology is letting many of us experience sexual pleasure that we wouldn't have access to otherwise.

Because doesn't everyone deserves to be all that *and* a bag of chips?

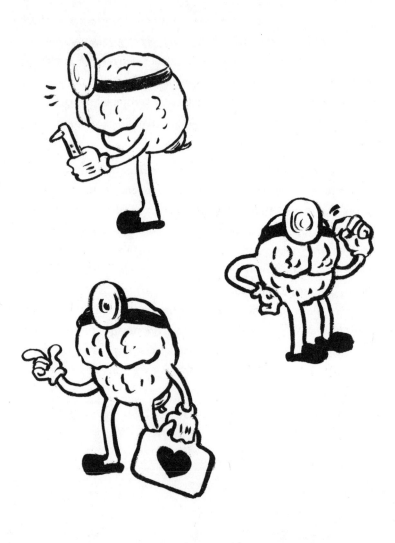

Sex Addiction and Porn Addiction Don't Exist

High sex drive, porn usage, masturbation, cheating, and other behaviors around sex have been increasingly attributed to sex addiction over recent decades. Sex addiction is a multi-billion dollar treatment industry … and it's based on something that literally doesn't exist.

I have *many* people come to see me because their behavior regarding sex or porn is really pissing off their partner. The word "addiction" starts getting thrown around, and the do-er gets an ultimatum that shit's over if they don't get therapy for their "problem."

Can you engage in sex (partnered or solo, porn-enhanced or not) in a way that is problematic? Sure. And we're gonna get into that. But there is one thing that needs to be said first: wanting sex, enjoying sex, and being excited about sex does not make you a sex addict. Having cheated on a partner means you did something shitty to someone you love, but it doesn't make you a sex addict. Wanting porn, enjoying porn, and being excited about porn does not make you a porn addict.

Let me say that one more time for the people in the back: *being sex and porn positive does not an addiction make.* Alfred Kinsey (hey there again, toothbrush dude!) once remarked, "A nymphomaniac is someone who has more sex than you do."

A therapist shouldn't diagnosis you with a sex or porn addiction, because the diagnosis doesn't exist in the DSM. And according to the research, there is simply no such thing.

Generally speaking, an addiction requires some physiological dependence for diagnosis. Problems with sexual activity tend to be labeled as a *process addiction*, which means there is no involvement of a substance that creates a literal physical dependency (like alcohol, nicotine, and other drugs), but the behavior itself has addictive qualities. When the brain lights up in the process of doing something like shoe shopping or gambling, it's easy to see the reward circuit being activated in a way it doesn't for someone who doesn't share that process addiction.

But sex (solo or partnered) is *supposed* to light up the reward centers of the brain. *Everyone's* brains light up that way. So can you safely label it an addiction? No. More research on better mechanisms for diagnosis are needed. But since we don't yet have a sex addiction blood test or brain scan test to rely on, figuring out problematic sexual behavior is individual and contextual. And it's one of those places where a well-trained, sex-positive therapist can be of benefit.

Can someone engage in sexual behaviors that harm their relationships and other life domains? Sure. But it is very important to call it what it really is. *Dismissing problematic behaviors as addiction is a denial of responsibility and a declaration of a lack of self-control.* And that right there is some fucking bullshit. Anyone who is engaging in problematic behavior around sex is absolutely accountable for their behavior and absolutely able to recognize their urges and consider how acting on them will impact their partners and their lives in general in the long term.

First of all, if you are worried that you may fall into the sex/porn problematic usage category, here are some questions to consider. But don't take your score as immutable evidence of your "addiction," okay? The point here is to discover patterns of behavior in order to create better strategies around the actions that are causing harm.

- Is partnered sexual activity itself more important than the person with whom you are having sex?

- Does the sexual activity take the place of true connection?

- Are you experiencing a lot of life stress right now? Or depression or grief or anything else that's really difficult to deal with, and have started using porn and/or sex more than usual as a coping skill?

- Are you skipping out on other important things in your life because of your behavior around sex and porn?

- Are you feeling out of control of your behavior, instead of seeing sex and porn as another way of expressing who you are as a person? Like, is it costing you money you don't have or causing legal or health consequences?

- Is sex or porn something you use for connection and/or fun, or is it a compulsion you fight with every day?

- Is your behavior at odds with what your partner thinks is appropriate? Your church? Your family? Your community? Is this about other people's core values or your own?

Here is the big thing I want you to look at: how sex and porn either hinder or support your relationships. In the end, all addictions are replacement relationships. They become more important than the people we love. They become more important than we are ourselves, and prevent us from being a human out there connecting in the world.

Problematic use of sex, masturbation, and/or porn comes about when the thing we are doing becomes more important than all of our reasons for being, and all of the meaning of our behaviors are drained of context. I don't know anyone who is unhappy with their usage of sex and/or porn who actually likes what they are doing. Not past the immediate moment of engagement, anyway. And they don't like themselves all too much, either. Because their behavior is separating them from all the amazing, messy, authentic, beautiful relationships the world has to offer, it's no longer aligned with their values and keeps them from prioritizing the people they love. That's what defines a problem.

If you are worried that your solo sex activities are problematic to your partnered sex (or if your partner states that they are), it's important to unpack the impetus of the behavior and the effect it's having on your other life domains. Generally speaking, when you are dealing with the other stressors in your life effectively, this "problem" takes care of itself.

If you realize that your current sexual activities are posing a problem for you, then it may be of benefit to get some support. One of the biggest problems in this area is the number of clinicians profiting on the stigma and shame surrounding sex. Which means that doing careful research is really important. Ask any therapists that you are interested in seeing what their stance on sex addiction and porn usage is. If you are dealing with past religious or cultural messages around your sex and pornography usage, ask them if they are comfortable with helping you explore that without adding their own value system to the conversation. I recently read an article by a therapist who views masturbation as a form of spousal abuse. Yes, literally. There is enough shame and stigma around sex out there as it is. You sure as fuck don't need it from your therapist.

PART THREE:
Unfuck Your
Relationship with Others

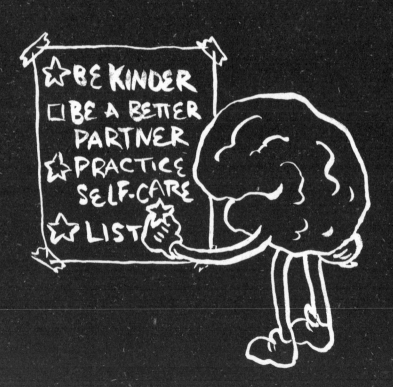

I s this the part of the book you were most interested in? Did you skip or skim the other stuff because you wanted to get to *this* stuff? Ok, go ahead and insert a big Kermit *yaaaaaaaaaayyyyyyyyy* right here. This is all the dating and relationshipping advice we could squeeze in, plus lots of activities to try. Fair warning though, I'm gonna refer back to the other two sections on occasion. So if you skipped them and emotional stuff comes up, you may have to head on back a few chapters and do some more unpacking!

My therapeutic training is grounded in relational-cultural theory. One of the biggest differences between this treatment orientation and others is that we regard relationships as their own entity. Meaning that in every connection we have with someone else, there is us, there is them, and there is the relationship itself as its own third party. This perspective is a bit of sorcery that can have an amazing impact on your romantic partnership.

So if Part Two of this book was the "you" part, this is the "relationship itself" part. And since you're a smart motherfucker, you noticed that I didn't include a "them" section. Because someone else is not your job, right? You are responsible for you. And you have a joint responsibility to the relationship. So we are focusing on you-in-relation here, not them. That's their job.

So this last part of the book includes far fewer naked shenanigans than you might expect. Because even if you are an exceptional specimen, only a small percentage of your time is actually spent on naked shenanigans. And all this other self-in-relationship stuff, like the communication and healthy boundaries, is the foundation for making that part far better.

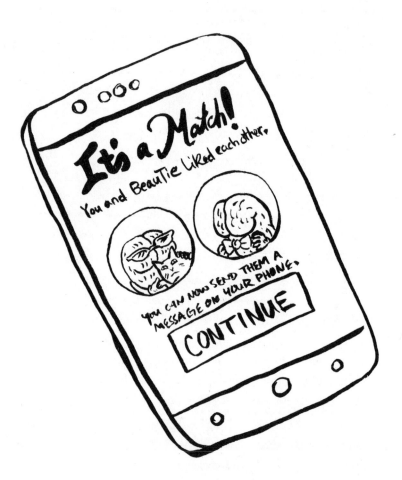

Date Like a Grown Up

D ating. What ever happened to *dating*? Wooing? Courting? Shaking your plumage and doing the mating dance?

There seems to be zero space these days between hooking up/friends-with-benefits and having the U-Haul number on speed dial. Either we make the beast with two backs and then take off *or* we move in and adopt a dog together in 3 minutes flat. Let's be honest, neither one is authentic. If sex without feelings has become your long-term solution, then you've fallen into the "it's cooler not to care" trap. It's safer there, you don't get hurt if it wasn't emotional to begin with. But belly flopping into something time after time isn't the more mature response. Then it becomes about being in a relationship, rather than being with a particular person with whom which you want to build a relationship. Desperate to connect is just as toxic, in the end, as desperate to stay disconnected.

Fuck. It's all pretty bonkers. The amount of time I have spent with clients and friends discussing the merits of different dating apps, local bars and hangouts, and other minutia of the dating scene is not a small number. Everything is a question: When do I start opening up about the heavy stuff? What's considered heavy stuff? When is too soon? When is too late? Why am I always friend-zoned?

No wonder we end up saying "fuck that noise" and settling in for another round of Candy Crush instead. Or end up spending years with someone who is not right for us, making each other miserable, because someone is better than no one, right? Dating becomes an obstacle course instead of what it is supposed to be, which is something *fun*.

Are you in that space? Early-stage almost-relationshipping? Considering the FTR (friends to relationship if you aren't fluent in acronym) move? Dating? Thinking about dating? Opening up the OKCupid website then feeling nauseous and closing the browser window immediately? Stressful as *balls*, isn't it?

I don't know about you, but I'm so over it. It's time for us to reclaim this space from the asshole culture around us. Roll up your sleeves, my blueberry muffins. Let's get to work.

How to Find a Date

It used to be we met the people we dated at school or church or because our parents arranged everything down to the number of goats everyone got out of the deal. Then the internet happened and shit changed. And generally for the better. Online chat rooms turned into IRL relationships and by 1995, the first official dating website (Match.com if you're interested) went live.

Instead of being limited to being only one or two degrees from Kevin Bacon, the whole world opened up and we connected with people completely outside our small social circles. Researchers from the University of Essex and University of Vienna were able to model the changes created by the advent of online dating. Currently, more than a third of marriages start with online dating. The number of interracial marriages has gone up significantly. Marriages born of meeting online are often stronger than those of people who meet in more traditional ways. The internet is the second most likely way someone who is heterosexual will find a partner, and it is far and away the most likely place for someone who is LBG+ to find someone to date.

That's not to say it's all well and good. Online dating can suck, too. The advent of swipe-apps (starting with Tinder in 2012) have made the process more game-like. You're essentially flipping through a card deck, creating accept and reject piles. And the process has fucked with a lot of people's self-esteem. Research presented at the American Psychological Association conference in 2012 demonstrated that people who used Tinder as a dating app had worse self-esteem than people who used other dating apps (going back to why self-compassion is so important, am I right??) and men specifically reported more negative body image perceptions than their counterparts on other sites.

So what's a modern human to do?

- If you are using a dating site, choose carefully. Think about your end goals (Marriage and all the baby-raising? Netflix and chill?) and pick a site that matches.

- Also, be honest about your end goals. Don't say you are good with keeping things casual when your reality is a ticking biological clock. And if you aren't sure, say that too. Maybe you are open to an LTR but that's not your immediate goal. If people self-select out because they want something different, then fine, that wasn't meant to be your person anyway.

- Be honest about all of it. Don't lie about your age, your weight, your circumstances. Seriously *stop* with the snap filter enhanced photos and the artful hand-under-the-chin tuck.

Look your best, but look yourself. And *be* yourself. Separated but not yet divorced? Own it. Have four kids? Own it. Polyam? Spill the details on what that means for you, your primary partner, other partners, and anyone you might date. Again, if people self-select out, they weren't meant to be your person anyway.

If online isn't your cup of tea, then you are gonna have to put yourself out there in other ways. Awkward and vulnerable, but far better than staying home and playing video games all weekend if what you actually want to do is meet someone. So you are gonna have to expand your social circle.

- Find people who are doing the interesting shit that you like to do. If tabletop gaming is your thing, join a meetup for gamers rather than just hanging out with your same crew all the time. If you're a jogger, join a running group. If you like movies and popcorn there are totally meetups just for people to get together to go the movies as a group. You may not meet the love of your life but at least you are doing something you enjoy and getting out of your regular circle. And maybe one of *those* people will end up introducing you to the love of your life at some point!

- Volunteer. If you are passionate about animal rescue or electing a particular candidate to office or anything else then volunteer to help make that happen. Just like with above, at least you aren't doing something that feels like a waste of time otherwise (fruitlessly hanging out a bar, anyone?), you will expand your social network, and you are racking up some bonus world-changing points in the process.

- Ask people who they know. Yeah, awkward. But if you want to go out with someone you gotta meet them first. You don't have to look for the Carrie Fisher in *When Harry Met Sally* friend who has a dude rolodex or anything, but just put it out there that you have an eye out, what you're looking for, and that you are amenable to an intro. And lest we forget? Carrie Fisher's character ended up marrying Bruno Kirby's character...and they met through Harry and Sally!

- Be prepared to approach in a way that is engaging but still authentic. Don't be the person in the coffee shop that interrupts someone who is reading or has headphones in. But if they're standing in line to order and are holding a book maybe try *"I keep seeing that book around* (or *I've never seen that book around*, whatever works)*—any good?"* as an opening line. You need a cold open? I have a friend who is not super-hot but has great game because he first approaches with *"Are you waiting on anyone?"* and if they say no, or say yes, but indicate it's a friend and not a date, he follows up with *"Is it cool if I flirt with you for a little while then?"* If you don't have the Sergeant Smooth gene, embrace your discomfort. The right person will think that's pretty cute. Maybe *"I'm gonna kick myself later if I didn't at least come up and introduce myself. And I'm feeling super awkward, so here's hoping I don't embarrass myself so badly that I will feel the urge to go walk into traffic. Hi, I'm..."*

- Make it your mission to start conversations with people in general so that approaching someone you think is super cute will seem less intimidating. Go practice!

Date Like a Therapist

Ok, so you met someone. The best dating advice i've got for ya? Date like a therapist.

I married early in my adult life while others my age were still dating. Then, in my late 30s, my husband died of cancer. Suddenly I was a young widow with two teenagers and a complicated career. The dating world had become a very different world since my years as a teenager. By the time I was ready to date I wasn't sure what awaited me. My specialty in private practice is intimacy and relationships. Would that complicate matters? Would I over-analyze everything and scare my dates away?

Instead, I found that the same qualities that made me a good therapist were of great benefit to dating. I was no longer in my early 20s, but neither were the men I met. Maturity was part of it, but an even more important factor was my therapeutic training. I didn't need to turn that part of myself off to enter the dating world; instead I found it to be very useful.

Eventually, I got married again, something I had no expectation of ever happening. I truly believe that dating like a therapist helped me find the man I am completely crazy about. and I wanted to share the benefit of these experiences with others in the dating market.

Be Present, Engaged, and Authentic

Most individuals give off certain signals demonstrating interest and availability in a dating environment. I was told by more than one person that I didn't send any of them. I didn't twirl my hair, giggle, or make extraneous physical contact on dates. One guy told me that at first he didn't know how to respond to me. He was used to gauging if someone was interested in him by reading these signals, but then he realized that he felt completely comfortable with me because I was focusing all my attention on him.

If I committed to a date with someone, even a meeting for coffee, I was committing my time and attention to that person. Everyone deserves the respect of an engaged and present response. My intent is to get to know the person, not put on a show for them. If someone comes to see me for therapy, they receive my undivided attention whether or not I find them interesting or likable. Dating someone should be the same. If I was too busy sending out flirty signals, I would miss getting to know someone in a truly authentic way.

Use SMART Goal Setting

When writing a treatment plan for a client, I ask the following questions to help formulate goals. Is the goal: Specific? Measurable? Achievable? Realistic? Time-Sensitive?

Dating should be no different. What do you want from your dating experience? How will you know if you are getting that? If you are looking for a life partner how will you know if you are on that path? If you are looking for someone to have fun with, what does fun look like for you?

Don't waste your time or theirs. Know what you want and how you plan on getting there. Consider where you are now and pay attention to any signals that suggest that your goals are changing. Not that wandering aimlessly is always a bad thing, but you are far more likely to get what you want if you know what that actually is.

Realize That Everyone Has Their Own Agenda

Much like someone walking into a therapist's office, anyone you are dating has their own agenda for their dating experience, an agenda that may or may not be congruent with your own. (The word agenda seems like a sinister one, I know. But in reality, it just refers to the motivations and intentions that we all carry into everything we do, including into our dating lives.) They may not even be fully aware of what they want. Not all agendas are explicit. Their hidden agendas may not have anything to do with you. Their motivations are not nearly as much about you as you think they are, so don't take everything personally.

I not only expect people to be guarded starting out in therapy, I *respect* it. If anything, dating is even more anxiety-provoking than starting therapy. So give both the other people and yourself some space. Be willing to explore, rather than make immediate demands. Relationship-building takes time, so give each potential new one space to grow.

Be Aware of Your Countertransference

Countertransference is a therapeutic word first coined by Freud in correspondence with Jung in 1909. He defined it as the therapist's emotional response to their client based on their own history or issues. Freud conceived this as a personal problem on the part of the therapist and something that should be guarded against and tamped down at all times.

More than 100 years later, we think about countertransference much differently. I teach my students that countertransference is entirely normal, and can be beneficial (as well as diagnostic) as long as we remain aware of it when it happens. This means parsing out whether other people have a similar response to this person, or just you. Essentially, the question becomes…when you have a strong emotional reaction to someone, it your stuff or theirs?

This is no different when dating someone new. If their behavior is upsetting or anxiety provoking in any way, listen for cues that other people have the same response to that person. This can lend insight into how they interact with others in general, and help you decide whether or not this is a behavior you want to endure.

On the other hand, if it seems to be just *your* response, then it is important that you do your own work around that, rather than expecting someone else to adapt to your triggers. Chances are, this will be something that will come up for you over and over again, even if you don't end up with this particular person, so you might as well do the work. We all have our own baggage in relationships, and it is important that we take responsibility for carrying it.

Know When to Terminate

"Firing" clients is a tough thing for a therapist to do. We struggle with knowing when it is appropriate and how to do so in the best possible way. This is where the SMART goal setting comes in. Are we progressing along the lines that we should be? Are we progressing at all? Is their agenda becoming more explicit? Can I adapt to the agenda and needs of the person I am seeing? Is the client showing up when they are supposed to and doing the things they said they are going to do?

Can you think of any better analogy for a break-up? I might be biased, but I never could.

The poet Maya Angelou was known for saying, "When someone shows you who they are, believe them." In the end, love is a behavior. Do you feel respected? Is your time valued? Do you feel the relationship is moving forward? If not, have you addressed these issues and asked for change?

I have told clients, "I don't think this is helping you and it is important that I don't waste your time. We either need to find a way to make this work or I can refer you to someone else." I have had similar conversations with people I have dated. Termination doesn't mean someone is a bad person. It means you are ending a bad match.

In the end, all of us deserve relationships that let us be our best possible selves, and support us in that endeavor. We need to know what we want, and give our relationships a chance to meet these desires. We also need to know when to let them go, or change the nature of them to better meet our needs. Therapy, in the end, should model what a health relationship can be like.

A therapeutic approach to dating can be a very effective strategy for creating the types of relationships we are seeking. It isn't your typical smoke and mirrors dating advice. Instead of hiding who you are, be exactly who you are—because that is the person you want others to see and know.

More Dating Tips for Grown-Ass People

My date-like-a-therapist advice was originally published by a local news organization and it was a hit. One of my bonus kiddos ended up getting it as a reading assignment in a class at the local community college, which cracked her up mightily. In the ensuing years, I've added other dating tips to the list based on the patterns I see happening with my clients, with my single friends, and even based on the *what-the-fucks* I think when reading shit online. So here's some more *taking the crazy out of dating* advice.

Have Fun. Yes. Seriously.

The fun part? That's the number one priority.

That doesn't mean don't be nervous. Because, duh, you likely will be. But at some point, you should be relaxing a bit and having a blast.

If you aren't busy picking out the names for your future children in your head, you can actually have fun. If you do an internal fun check and you aren't thinking "I'm digging this person! Woohoo!" then nothing is there for you. That's okay. A date is just a date. Far less serious and heart-wrenching if it ends with just that.

Do a Deep-Down Gut Check

Does something feel off? Unsafe? Listen to that. Listen *hard*. If your intuition tells you that something is fundamentally wrong at any point, don't ignore it. This is so difficult for people who have spent their lives being silenced and being told that what they think and feel doesn't matter. You may have been told for so many years about the wrongness of your instincts that you have trained yourself to stop listening to them. Dating is the time to listen again. Get down in your gut and see what it's telling you. Did you know the vagus nerve connects the brain and stomach? We really do, at a literal level, have a second brain in our stomachs. Listen to it.

Beyond the gut check, do the spark check. Do you get the little pitter-patter when you brush someone's arm or during that first kiss? You deserve pitter patter. Maybe there's no pitter-patter because you are super nervous or maybe it's because you really aren't feeling it. It's okay if you're not. Pay attention to that.

Everyone Deserves to Be Chocolate Cake

I had a client tell me that his partner of 30+ years still makes his heart skip a beat. That's amazing. We all deserve to feel that for someone and be that for someone. If you are dating a person who is amazingly fantastic but doesn't pass the fun check and the spark check, you don't have to keep digging for it. It's okay to think someone is amazing but have zero interest in seeing them naked.

They can be a great person, but not a great person for you. The important thing is that *you tell them that*.

I dated my way to a lot of great friendships. It's not an easy conversation, but it doesn't have to be a complicated one. Be honest. Say something like *"This may sound like bullshit but I mean every word when I say I think you're amazing and totally deserve someone who thinks you hung the moon and I'm not going to be that person. I don't want you out of my life, but I respect it if me not wanting to date you anymore means you'd rather not see me at all."* This is better for everyone in the long run, even if it feels awful in the short run. If they get butthurt at your disinclination to sexitimes with them and don't want to remain friends, that's okay, too.

You also should be aware of your own patterns in this regard. Do you find you always get bored pretty quickly with genuinely nice people who aren't creating a level of chaos energy that keeps things exciting (but still ultimately toxic)? Did all your relationship models function on drama and dysfunction? Do you tend to have three week stands and then wander off to the next big thing? Chocolate cake doesn't require crazy sprinkles to be yummy. If you are realizing that about yourself, maybe it's time to go back to Parts One and Two and do some work on yourself, yeah?

Beware the Oxytocin Trap

Oxytocin is the love drug… the neurochemical best known as *Wheeeeeeeeeeeeeeeeeeee*! Oxytocin is released in physical touch (and yes, *especially* in orgasms). And it's *awesome*. But it can also be an asshole. We call it the love drug, but it's really the trust drug. It makes us feel like we can trust the person we are with far more than we likely would otherwise. This is why a salesperson will touch your arm when trying to get you to close a deal. This is also why if you go all-in on a new relationship it will burn out fast.

If you are with a new person 24/7, you never get a break from the oxytocin flood to actually do a good gut check. Kinda like Kilgrave's hold on his victims in season one of Jessica Jones. Make space away from them to see how you feel. Are you halfway-relieved when they aren't around? Do you feel better about yourself without them there? Less on guard? Why is that? Do you miss them? What do you actually miss? Are they being shitty about you taking time and space for yourself? Are they pressuring you to be present when you aren't? Does that make you feel controlled? This goes back to the gut check questions. It's important to pay attention to how the trust drug may impact our answers and lead us astray, so you may need to make space for yourself to answer them better.

Don't Make Your Friends and Family Ride Your Drama Llama With You

If you tend to live in the land of one week stands, that's your decision. Dragging everyone along with you is a pretty dick move, however. Even if you don't have a new person in place on the reg, it's important to live your life, not your new relationship.

My general rule of thumb is if you are out with your other people, spend about 25% of your time talking about your new person and 75% of the time talking about *all the rest of your life*. It's important to remember that you have one and it's important not to irritate the fuck out of the people around you. Your new relationship is important, too. I get it. But is it 100% of everything you say important? Nah, 25% is plenty.

The people who I've seen working out in the long term are the ones that are out living their lives, not dissecting every move every single minute. What is going on that you feel the need to do a critical incident stress debriefing over every text? Is this something about you that you need to work on, or something about the relationship? If you are feeling so unsettled with this new person that you are having to water-cooler quarterback every play? Something is up. Maybe with you, if that's your pattern. And if it is? Work on that shit. But if you are generally Captain Chill? Gut check this thing.

Consider Stepping Back a Bit on Having Your Friends Meet Each New Person

Give it at least a month. My general rule was 3-4 months. And if you have kids? More like 6 months. And if this new person is pressuring you otherwise? Ask them (and yourself) *why?* If they aren't going anywhere, then they aren't going anywhere. They don't have to be dumped full force into your life to prove anything.

Look for Slippage

There is something about that four-month mark, I swear. We can hold ourselves together and show our best sides for about that long, tops. Then our authentic self starts leaking out around the edges. Keep an eye out for boo-person's real personality to start showing up. This isn't a bad thing. In fact, a lot of idiosyncrasies can be downright adorable. Like Friday night pancakes for dinner or leaving the Sunday paper on the floor because the cat loves to sleep on it. Some things aren't great but are tolerable, and are important to know about someone, like low blood sugar hanger, irritability in traffic, that kinda thing.

Some things may need to be deeply considered and discussed: Rudeness to waitstaff. Disinterest in voting in elections. A deep and abiding love of Nickelback. You know, seriously important, possibly deal-breaking shit.

When I asked friends for their dating rules, one said "Don't date… interrogate." Another said, "Talk to one another until dawn at least three times." Again, no matter how much you think you know this person's soul after a couple of weeks, you don't. And no matter how much you think they know *you*, they really, really don't. Oxytocin is a fucking liar. Take the time to have those deep conversations and really get to know someone.

Don't Give Your Power Away

A friend of mine said, in regard to dating, "Never treat them like a priority if they only treat you like an option." Another said, "Want what you want for yourself (love, connection, desire) more than you want any one person." This may seem like two separate pieces of advice, but it really isn't. Both people, in their way, are saying, don't give your power away.

Anyone you are with should enhance your life, enhance your hopes and dreams, and enhance your compassion and engagement with yourself and the world around you. Someone who is not excited about you and about what you bring into the world isn't worth your time.

A Rejection May Not Have a Damn Thing to Do With You

If all your relationships end at date number three, it may be time to figure out what is happening there, either in your behavior or in the people you are choosing. But generally speaking? If you are dating someone and you get a big ole swipe left? That is far less about you then you realize. Seriously. Someone you asked out? Or you've been out with them a couple times? They don't know you well enough to reject the actual awesomeness that is you.

They are rejecting your *offer* for getting to know the real, awesome you. For whatever reason. Maybe their ex called. Maybe they don't like your choice of band t-shirts. Maybe they are oxytocin junkies off in search of their next hit. Maybe they are stupid motherfuckers who don't know a good thing when it is standing right in front of them. But, hey. You haven't had the deep getting to know each other conversations for you to take this rejection all kinds of personally. Dating doesn't magically lead to relationshipping. It isn't supposed to. It's supposed to be a try out period. Next candidate!

Date Safely and Have a Disclosure Plan

There are all kinds of things we may need to disclose to a new dating partner. Things that are not any of the business of other people in our life but could affect an intimate relationship. That we are unemployed and broke AF. That we have kids. That we are poly or into kink. That we have an STI. Information about our gender identity or sexual orientation.

If you have something big that can affect relationships, it's really important to have a disclosure plan. And sometimes the information you are disclosing can put you at risk with the other person (and/or anyone they tell). If your truthbomb conversation runs the risk of ending very badly, also have a safety plan: Have the conversation in a public place, have a friend on stand-by, and have an escape plan.

I can tell you as a rule of thumb, I generally go with *"lay it all on the table and let people self-select out if it's a problem."* If this is presented immediately, there is less need for big disclosure sessions later. And yes, I totally get that people will self-select out that would have been great partners if they had gotten to know you first. But I am not that invested in developing the emotional maturity of people I don't know and may or may not end up liking. And just looking at the number of trans women of color who are victims of intimate partner violence makes me desperate to encourage all y'all to err on the side of caution and keep yourself safe in the long run.

Many of my clients have decided to use dating sites that are specific to their situation for just this reason. There are sites for individual who have STIs, who are trans, who are poly, who are into BDSM, who are into roleplay. There is legit an app for all the different kinds of ways we can be a human in relationships.

Some things on the "need to disclose" list may have legal consequences if you don't handle it right. For example, knowingly transmitting an STI to a new, uniformed partner could get you into legal trouble. I live in Texas, where some STIs could carry the weight of an assault charge and others (namely, HIV and AIDS) could find you charged with attempted murder or assault with a deadly weapon.

But, hey. I'm not a lawyer. This is not legal advice. And legal shit aside, telling people the truth is just the right fucking thing to do. So *disclose.* Before you don't-disclose to someone who finds out, freaks out, dumps you, tells the world, *and* maybe even presses charges.

You Are Allowed to Be Crazy, You Aren't Allowed to Act Crazy
I have said this so many times, I need to get a tattoo at this point. Whatever nutty things are running through your mind? Don't act on them.

Yes, you have baggage. We all do. If you know your past history has messed up your thinking about relationships, then you need to work on that shit and not foist it upon the people you are dating. Emotions are just information from our body—whatever you feel isn't right or wrong. But your actions are your responsibility. If you know that doing something will embarrass you later, do not do the thing.

What's the thing, you ask innocently? Different for different people. But we all have a pair of big, striped crazy pants hidden in the backs of our closets. And we all feel the urge to dig them out, put them on, and act all kinds of stupid over relationship issues. It may be driving by their house to see who is parked there, setting up a fake Facebook account to stalk them, or getting color contacts so your eyes match. Whatever weirdness your brain is telling you is a good idea? Don't do it.

If you know you will look back on the situation and realize you were wearing your big striped crazy pants that day? *Do not do the thing.* Get a friendervention. Hide your phone and car keys from yourself. Don't lash out. Don't be reactionary. You are responsible for yourself and whatever baggage you still carry (no matter who packed those bags to begin with). Hold yourself accountable.

Be Wise

This piece of advice was given to me by Joe McBride (yes, of *Rock 'n' Roll High School* fame). If you haven't read his memoir, *The Broken Places,* you really should. If you have, you know he has some intense and dark relationships. When I asked him what he meant by "be wise," he responded, "It's like when Gertrude Stein was dying, and Alice B. Toklas said, 'Gertrude, Gertrude, what is the answer?' Gertrude replied, 'What is the question?'"

I know, academics tell the most esoteric jokes. Joe was really saying, be wise in whatever ways make sense for you, your needs, and your relationships. Shift based on what you need to shift. Be aware enough of your own shit to know where you need to be careful. Listen to your instincts. Believe what people show you more than what they tell you. Be thoughtful. Consider *all* the ways they are communicating with you. People are always telling their stories and sometimes they even use words. This kind of attention to the world around us is how we can be wise.

On The Glories of *Not* Dating (And Maybe Even Still Having Sex!)

You don't have to be in one of the ace/demi/gray/aro categories to not be interested in dating. After all, you can have plenty of sex, solo or partnered, without ever dating, right?

It usually boils down to a few basic reasons:

1) You've got shit you are actively working on so you can be a good human being in relation to other human beings.

2) You are way too fucking busy with other shit to add more shit to your plate. You can't focus on it, you don't have the time, and you don't want to be dickish to someone else in the process of you finishing school, working crazy hours, raising kids, etc.

3) You just aren't that into it. You're happy and fulfilled and dating doesn't add anything to the mix for you at this time in your life.

All of these reasons are excellent ones. And you are totally entitled to not-date to your single-lovin' heart's content. But hey, if you are not-dating because of anxieties or other reasons when the truth is you really, really actually want to date? It isn't the worst idea in the world to upack what's holding you back. Therapy can help with that. You deserve to be happy, and if dating will help you get there, let's figure that shit out.

Are you not-dating but still wanting some partnered-sex game? Also totally fine. Despite how progressive culture has gotten in so many ways, we still manage to get our prude on about no-strings sex. There is zero wrong with having an FWB or pick ups and hookups. If that's what works for you, go for it. Just as long as everyone is on the same page about the plan. It should probably go without saying that you need to be careful about preventing STIs and unwanted pregnancies and the like. But you're a responsible person and you know that, right?

You may notice that your level of sexual satisfaction is not as good with partners you don't have an emotional attachment to. Research says that's generally the case. That's not me saying you should be all boo'd up with anyone you have sex with. But there *is* a reason the expression is *friends with benefits*. The friends part is legit important for most people. As a general rule, if you wouldn't vote for someone if they were running for public office, letting them have naked sexitime isn't something you are going to feel great about in the grander scheme.

Of course, all this can lead to the problem of someone in the hook-up relationship catching feelings. It's not a bad thing or an embarrassing thing. But it is something that needs to be discussed and dealt with. Which goes back to the full disclosure dialogue. Not a fun conversation, but a needful one. Even just *"I know this is supposed to be low-key, but lately I've been wanting it to be more. If you do too, that would be amazing and we should talk about that.*

If not, I probably need to not see you since it's gonna mess with my head and I don't wanna go all crazy on the both of us."

No matter what your circumstances, keep it honest and watch for your own motivations and reactions. You won't always do everything perfectly, but you are far less likely to be blindsided that way.

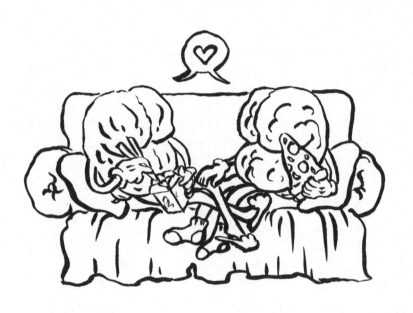

Relationshipping

R elationshipping is not dating. And thank Buddha, because even if you are going in with the healthiest attitude ever, dating can be really tiring.

Of course, getting boo'd up has its own set of crap to navigate. In some ways you are safer and more secure and you don't have to worry so much anymore. But on the other side, I see folx feeling *too* safe and secure and unworried, and then fuck things up cuz you go in all Leeerrrrrooooooooy Jennnnnkiiiiiiiins style. And I don't want that for you. You've been working too hard on all this shit to biff out now.

A relationship is always ongoing work. Especially for those of us who didn't have great role models in that regard and have to be proactive in our desire to be healthier in our relationships than what we saw around us growing up. Whether you and your partner are still all new and shiny, or whether you have years under your belt, actively working on your relationship in the small ways will make the larger obstacles far easier to deal with (and may end up preventing them all together).

I realize that most of these rules aren't about sex at all…which makes sense because the book is called *Unfuck Your Intimacy*, not *Unfuck Your Fuck*. These are all guidelines and ideas for improving intimacy generally, which will improve physical intimacy in turn.

Love People, Not Labels

Boy or girl. Neurosurgeon or flight attendant. Labels are assignments we attach to aspects of our being. They are not the sum entirety of who we are. And they change. They change all the time. So if you become attached to the label that someone wears, you are going to be sadly disappointed when that label falls off. The only label your partner should ever get from you? "Mine."

Grow together and put one another first

The strongest relationships I see are the ones that go through enormous changes together. In physical ability, career, socio-economic status, even gender.

How do you marry someone you thought was a man and be in their process of realizing they are a woman? Stay with them through all their gender confirmation treatments and surgeries even if your own sexual orientation never included women? Loving that person like a motherfucking *boss*, that's how.

When long-term relationships start to fall apart over longer periods of time, it's often because partners don't remain connected in their growth. People change. *All the time.* Life changes us, maturity changes us, and our circumstances put us in places we never thought we'd be. Losing sight of our partner as our primary person in this world happens most often when we have children. But other things can cause this to be an issue as well. Careers, other family, friends. Your partner may have interests that are wildly different from your own, or interests that you never expected.

Unless we are with people who are harming themselves or others, they deserve support. Be your partner's biggest cheerleader and expect them to be yours. Knowing that a person you choose to spend your life with is right behind you, keeping an eye on your six for you, is the best feeling in the world.

And then, together, as a team, go tackle the world. Have you heard the term "yoke" before? It's an old-fashioned word, used to describe the crossbeam that was used to connect two farm animals together so they could effectively pull a plow. And no, I'm not calling you an ox or a cow. It became a term to later explain marriage. The idea is that two equal partners, organized to work together can accomplish way more than two separate individuals. We work harder, stronger, and more effectively as a yoked team.

If you have kids, put each other first and then as a team put the children first. Or whatever else you are tackling. You and your partner must come first to each other. To keep from flying off in different directions and working toward different ends, stay yoked.

Spend Time Together

And I don't mean collapsed on the sofa, watching Netflix and eating ice cream in your stained sweats with boo by your side. I mean real, planned couples time. Your mate deserves to be wooed. And so do you.

This doesn't mean fancy, it just means intentional. It doesn't matter if it's a walk in the park, ice cream cones, or eating take-out and streaming the movie you missed in the theater. The point is respecting your relationship enough to make time for it in the same way you make time for everything else of importance in your life. Do you make an appointment when you go see your dentist? Plan in your schedule to run to Trader Joe's for groceries? Isn't boo (and hey, *all* of them if you have more than one) worth at least as much consideration?

Make a plan. To do something. Together. Once a week. It can even be at home if that is how life is rolling right now. But make that plan.

Spend Time Apart

This is stupid important if you and boo share a living space. And *especially* if you have kids. Once a week you should each have a chance to escape the house alone and once a week you should have a chance to have the house to yourself alone. I know how hard this is to do, but if you make effort to make the alone time happen, you will hit the mark more often than you are hitting it now, right?

It doesn't have to be complicated. Doesn't matter if you want to go wander Target with a Starbucks in hand for an hour alone; we all need time that is just ours. Same with time alone in the house. Doesn't matter if you do laundry and watch *Mozart in the Jungle* with the cat. The house. Alone. No judgments on how you spend that time. It's all yours. We all need that time to reboot, recharge, and be good partners.

Establish Your Relationship "Rules"

Everyone's relationship is different, which means everyone needs a structure to support their relationships. We call this structure "rules" for lack of a better term, though most of us have enough anarchist in us to hate the idea of rules. Scaffolding Of Interpersonal Respect work better? Use whatever feels right...but no matter what you call it? *Use your fucking words to communicate your expectations.* Whether we label it a want, a need, a boundary, etc., if there is an expectation you have of your partner? Y'all need to have that discussion.

Picture it. My office. Any time, because it happens at least once a week:

Partner 1: *They didn't.......[mad, mad, hurt, upset, grump, grump, complain]*

Partner 2: *....*

Me: *Did Partner 2 know you expected them to do that?*

Partner 1: *They should have!*

Me: *I see. Did you TELL them you expected that?*

Partner 1: *No! They should know!*

Me: *I flunked Mind-Reading School. I'm guessing Partner 2 did as well. Can you share with both of us what your expectations are so Partner 2 has a shot of getting out of trouble here?*

Partner 2: *I woulda been fine with doing what you wanted. But I'm concrete as pavement. Please tell me!*

Remember earlier when I said no one in the history of ever has run toward their lover in slow motion across a field of flowers. There isn't anything "natural" or "intuitive" about understanding someone else. Some people are good guessers, but if you really want to be understood then you better state shit up front. That's relationship rules in a nutshell.

Expect flowers on your birthday? Say it.

Expect Boo to not chat with exes on Snapchat? Say it.

Expect to meet all potential secondary partners before their first date? Say it.

Expect oral sex on Sunday afternoons? Sayyyyy the thing.

Once it's all out in the open, then you can sift through the disagreements. And bring in a therapist if you hit an impasse. But it's not rocket science. It's adulting. Which requires vulnerability and clear communication. And it isn't movie-romantic. Because we aren't living in a movie. And as uncomfortable as it is, it's better than cleaning up the damage caused by NOT having these conversations.

Everyone Has the Right to Feel Safe

We have the right to physical safety and emotional safety. Physical safety doesn't just mean free from interpersonal violence, it means feeling in control of your personal body at all times. I've worked with people who have never laid a hand on their partner, but they have a way of dominating with their physical presence that feels threatening and intimidating. That can be an intentional way of controlling the other person, and it is not safe or acceptable.

Emotional safety can be equally hard to define. I ask people to describe the sensations in their body when they feel a sense of safety. Not just their thoughts and feelings, but how they settle into themselves. Like how we feel when we crawl into a comfortable bed with soft sheets at the end of a long day. The people in our lives should support that feeling inside us, and we should do the same for them whenever we can.

Don't Fucking *Lie*

Don't half-truth. Don't omit. Don't answer on a technicality, Captain Semantics. Own your shit. Be honest and be authentic. Own it as yours but *say it*. If you are angry say you are angry, take responsibility and say why, ask for something different and hope you will get it. But don't say you are okay when you are not. And FFS, don't play a semantics game in your mind. Don't be sneaky. Don't be sketch. Don't rationalize. If your partner would be legitimately hurt or upset by anything they saw in your phone or on your computer, don't fucking do it.

Don't Kick the Puppy

Don't allow yourself bad behavior, even if your partner does. If you kick a puppy, it may come back and lick your hand over and over again. But that is not an excuse to keep kicking. If you know your actions are hurting your partner at some level, you have to stop. Even if they say it's okay. Even if they are not brave or strong enough to ask you to stop. Have some self-accountability. Stop the behavior or get out of the relationship.

This seems to happen in relationships where one partner is not chocolate cake. If one partner has all the power in the relationship because their mate is slavishly devotional in keeping them happy and keeping them there, a lot of metaphorical puppy kicking takes place. Taking advantage of their desperation, blowing them off at the last minute, accepting gifts and favors, messing around when they didn't agree to polyamory, generally being rude and disrespectful. Just because someone lets you treat them like that does not mean its ok. You've heard of the golden rule right? Even better? The platinum rule. Treat others the way they want to be treated. If you can't do that for your partner, or you don't want to, you need to move on.

Love Is a Behavior, Not a Feeling

Love is not a nebulous idea. It's not a vague notion of warm and fuzzies. It's the real, daily interactions of sharing our lives with someone, caring for them, and having them care for us in return. Love is what we *do*, day in day out. Not what we profess in our status updates.

Love is stopping what you are doing to sit with your mate and talk about their bad day. It's making sure they have avocados in the fridge for their favorite snack. Love is making time for date night even when you've been together for years and decades. Love is sending a text saying "I was just thinking about you, how's your day? Love you." It's living our lives with this person at our side at all times, even if they aren't physically present.

Be a More Excellent You

Do you know what rocks? You not expecting a mate to fix everything wrong in your life and doing that shit yourself. Because when you are a jacked-up mess, your bat signal attracts the same. Actively working on your shit is excellent advice whether you are single or already partnered.

No one says you have to be perfect. Mr. Dr. Harper loves me for my flabby belly and scrawny butt. Not because he finds them empirically sexy (but to each their own if that's your thang), but because they are attached to someone who has worked hard to build a life we are excited about. We are both people with goals we go after with full force. We take responsibility for our fuck-ups and help each other be better people. This may mean never trusting him to take the trash out in the morning no matter how much he swears he won't forget. But hey, healthy doesn't mean flawless.

I have had clients come see me after being so fucking tired of ruining relationship after relationship because they hadn't worked on their own shit. And it's so cool to see them do that work and then, at some point, tell me with enormous surprise that they met someone amazing and are building a great relationship. "I told them about my history and they stuck around." Of course they did. Because your history stopped defining you. And they know they are dating a human being who is working on their own shit.

You deserve someone great. And they deserve someone as great as you. Yes you have baggage. Your job is to carry your own rather than expect someone else to show up with a trolley.

Fuck All the Rules

All the ideas. All the guidelines. All of them. Even these ones if they don't fit. I mean, I can't see why...I think they're excellent. But you know what? You and your partner need to make your own map. Hell, maybe even partner isn't the right word. Maybe you are polyamorous and "partners" is the better word. You do you.

If you and your partner are delighted with the course you have charted, keep staying true. Keep the dialogue open, make corrections as needed, and love each other silly.

AGGRESSIVE

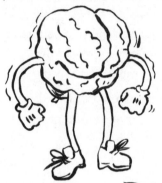

ASSERTIVE

PASSIVE

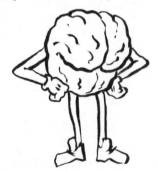

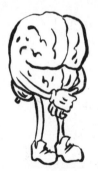

Unfuck Your Communication

Man. Relationships are kind of a dick move when you think about it. Our partners see the absolute worst side of us when they are the people we love best and who love us best. We are nicer to the bratty toddler running through the aisles at Target than we are to boo, who has seen us upchuck at 3 a.m., smelled our morning breath, and cleaned our pee off the toilet seat.

It's human nature to be toughest on the people we are closest to. This is why we tend to pick fights with our mate more than with anyone else.

When someone is your partner you have to constantly negotiate and navigate boundaries. And it's an ongoing process. Relationships are fluid entities that are always morphing and reshaping themselves as we live in them. But what really needs to be navigated? And when can you just let boo be boo?

If our boundaries are the essential building blocks of our relationships, then how we communicate these boundaries is critical. So many of our relationship fights could have been headed off at the pass if we had communicated proactively to begin with. I know I've been guilting of nurturing a world of butthurt that would have been easily prevented if I had just used my words. Unless you are a total specimen of perfection, you've probably done the same at some point. Changing how we engage can make all the difference in the world. And if the fight happens anyway? We got skills for that, too.

Communication Styles

Understanding how we communicate is the first step in actually communicating. Generally speaking, we aren't taught how to do so, so we have to figure that part out first.

There are three main styles:

Aggressive communication styles tend to be excessively harsh. Aggressive communicators tend to interrupt others, disregard others' opinions, and continually reinforce their own worldview and "rightness." Have you ever met anyone like this? Seen a politician on TV act like this? You know the type. You say you like pineapple on pizza and they roll their eyes and tell you that's gross, you're wrong, and you need to stop. *The meta-message of aggressive communicators is "I'm cool and you're a dumbass."*

Assertive communication style is our sweet spot in most cases (unless your literal safety is on the line and being situationally aggressive makes sense). Assertive communicators are firm in their belief systems and speak in a way that is congruent with their actions. But they do so in a way that still respects differing viewpoints. If you say you want pineapple on your pizza, they may respond with "Glad to see you out there living your best life. I've heard y'all pineapple pizza folx exist. Pineapple on your half of the pie it is. Get pineapple juice on my half, though, and I may hafta cut you." *The meta-message of assertive communicators is "I'm cool and you're totally cool, too. Even if we don't agree."*

Passive communication style tends to be ineffective in helping people protect themselves and hold their center. Passive communicators often don't make their wants and needs known, and say that things are fine when they are really, totally, deeply not fine. Passive communicators tend to defer to others, praising them while dumping on themselves. This isn't the same thing as letting someone you know and trust help guide you to better decision-making in a crisis. This is about never feeling like you can authentically advocate for what is right for you. Passive communicators, back to the pizza example I apparently cannot let go of, might say "Oh, pineapple. That would definitely be the better choice. Let's do pineapple. I can use hydrocortisone for the rash it gives me. Yeah, I'm allergic. But not really bad. It's totally okay." *The meta-message of passive communicators is "I'm a hot mess, but you're totally cool, so you make the decisions for both of us."*

Some questions to reflect on:

- What is your general communication style most of the time? Is that different in different circumstances or with different people?
- What messages have you internalized about your right to healthy communication and ownership of your values and beliefs?
- If you communicate differently in certain situations, or with certain people, what about those relationships causes you to change?
- How close is your current communication style to what your ideal balance would be?
- What is the first place you can start to shift your communication style, moving closer to your ideal? How will you go about doing that?

If you don't communicate as well as you would like to, owning that is really important.

As in, *"Hey partner-person! I realized recently that I don't communicate things that are important to me nearly as well as I should. Then I end up butthurt because you didn't understand what I was trying to say and you end up confused AF, which is understandable. I'm working on that. So what I've been trying to say, albeit, not well, is…"*

If you have this conversation, I'm totally awarding you a gold star for badass adulting.

The biggest thing to remember here that it is a process. You may need to ask each other questions and keep figuring things out. You may have to clarify what you mean until it comes out right. Your partner may resist the entire conversation (which means you have an entirely different issue). This ain't easy shit.

Communicating Like a Grown Person

Learning to communicate more assertively and effectively doesn't require a weekend Tony Robbins retreat. It just means considering effective communication as a skill, learning that skill, and practicing until it becomes second nature.

Do you remember the Pythagorean theorem? You totally just recited "a squared plus b squared equals c squared" in your head, didn't you? Did you ever use that outside of school? Yeah, me neither. You know what would have been way more helpful to learn? How to communicate with "I statements."

Try this with your partner when you are all kinds of hacked off (or all kinds of thrilled, for that matter):

> I feel _____
>
> when you _____ .
>
> What I want is _____ .

You know what this is? Being a grown-ass person who takes responsibility for their own feelings and actions and clearly communicates their needs, rather than blaming boo ("You made me mad!") or doing the freeze-out-no-talking thing ("If you really loved me you would read my mind!").

It's gonna feel all kinds of weird and awkward at first. I've had lots of people tell me that they bust out laughing the first few times they try it. It's just so *unnatural*, isn't it? Because we don't encourage people to talk like this, taking accountability and responsibility for their feelings.

But we *should*.

Our feelings are completely our own, and we shouldn't blame others for them. We can, however, ask them for different behaviors that better respect our boundaries. This skill works in regular communication and stays in place even if your convo has leveled up to conflict level. Staying with ownership of your own feelings completely shifts away from the blame game.

You can even take an extra step in acknowledging that they didn't intend the distress you felt, for instance by adding:

I felt uncomfortable when you made that joke just now. I know you just meant it to be funny and thought I would laugh rather than be upset. But I struggle with jokes about that topic. I would really appreciate it if you didn't tell jokes like that around me.

That's awesome shit right there. And bonus points on this, because boo can't tell you how to feel if you are taking ownership of it. It's not right or wrong, it's just what you feel. Adulting FTW.

Troubleshooting Your Communication

We are all trying to communicate mo' better. Communicating with the "I statements" model is a great strategy for being more mindful of that process. But figuring out where the breakdowns come from the most often is also hugely beneficial. I first heard this model in an online course I was streaming on Neuro-Linguistic Programming. I can't find a reference to it anywhere, so I don't know the origin story (and if you do, please drop me a line). Discussing an idea without the appropriate citation and attribution upsets my little academic heart, but it's too brilliant to not share.

The basic idea is that each exchange of verbal dialogue has four levels:

1) *What we mean to say.* You know, the actual idea you are trying to express.

2) *What we actually say.* If you are really good at only saying exactly what you mean at all times, I hope you write a book on your technique. For us regular humans, what we have in our minds and what comes out of our mouths is not always a solid match.

3) *What the other person hears.* Just because you said it doesn't mean they heard it without any filter.

4) *What the other person thinks you mean.* Even if you said "anything for dinner is fine" and you *meant* anything for dinner is fine, your partner may think there is a hidden agenda, or other things going on beyond the words that actually came out of your mouth.

Every couple I have worked with who is struggling with a communication breakdown has a problem in at least one of these areas. Generally, we are high achievers and are activating more than one if not all of them. Figuring out where the breakdown is informs the strategies to repair it.

Let's go back to the often-contentious decision about what to have for dinner:

1) *What you mean to say.* Maybe growing up, you weren't allowed to voice much opinion. Maybe you tend to think your answers are wrong. Maybe you get up in your head about what you want and get paralyzed when trying to communicate. If you don't express yourself well (or aren't great at figuring out what you want), being more measured and considered before responding can make a huge difference. Dinner example? It's okay to say, "Good question, let me think a minute," then actually check in on yourself. Maybe you genuinely *don't* care. Or maybe you really do want pizza and should say that.

2) *What you actually say.* Here is where you gotta use your words. Instead of "[mumble, mumble] like, pizza? Or maybe tacos if that's what you want. Chinese food? Um, there's soup left in the fridge…" say the truth. Like, "I've been jonesing for deep dish all day" or "I had tacos at lunch so anything other than Mexican food sounds good." Clear communication means that partner-person doesn't have to figure out which answer is the correct one.

3) *What the other person hears.* We all have our own interpretations, filters, and distractions. For this example, let's say partner-person hears the "I had tacos for lunch" part of your answer but not the "anything other than Mexican food sounds good" part and suggests fajitas for dinner. Do a gentle correction. If it's a continued problem and you are discussing bigger issues than dinner plans, it might help to ask your partner to repeat back in their words what you just told them. As in "I heard you say…"

4) *What your partner thinks you mean.* So many people have had past relationships where all responses were a death trap, they were supposed to mind read and interpret everything that was told to them, and there was hell to pay if they didn't. If you have a partner who over-interprets what you say, they may benefit from a reminder that you are responsible for your responses, and they don't have to mind-read. If you say "anything for dinner is fine" and you really mean "pizza" you better fucking say pizza, or not bitch when you get tacos for two meals in a row, right?

Resolving Conflict

Even the world's best communicators still have conflict. If the goal was never to have conflict, that would be easy. You would just have to be a total doormat and give people whatever they want all the time. If you don't want to be a doormat, the goal isn't conflict avoidance, but conflict management.

When things go sideways in your relationship, consider the following questions and strategies:

Is It Intentional?

Is your partner intentionally fucking with you? Like deliberately disrespecting your time, resources, needs, and desires? Like, *"I know we had dinner plans but I went out drinking instead because fuck you"*?

You have every right to be mad. But also? What the *actual, literal hell are you doing with this person*? If they have no fucks to give about what's important to you, get *out*. Believe what they are showing you about who they are. Call your bestie to request sofa surfing privileges, pack up your pooch, polish your tiara, and move on.

Fighting is worthless here. Because you are being treated like *you* are worthless here. Don't fight with someone who has made it clear that they don't care.

Who You Really Mad at, Cupcake?

Remember learning about Freud's defense mechanisms in Psych 101? He may have snorted too much coke, but he was right on about that shit. Displacement is a defense mechanism where we attack the safe target rather than the real cause of distress. Of course you can't tell your boss that his mother was a hamster and his father smelt of elderberries. So you get home already riled up and ready to rumble. Boo tells you they forgot to pick up your dry cleaning and you find yourself spewing venom like a champ.

If you know you are ripe for a fight, like after a hard day, do what you need to do to decompress that doesn't involve sniping at partner-person. And warn them that you are wound tight. It's totally okay to say a discussion needs to be put in the parking lot for the rest of the day, just tell your partner that's on you. Something to the end of "I'm so upset I'm afraid I'll be hurtful or mean in ways that I don't really feel. And I know I won't communicate well right now. I'm gonna go soak in the tub and figure out why I'm so upset, because I don't think this is all about you. Can we talk about this later?" The big thing is actually setting a date for later—don't use that as a sidestep technique to never have difficult conversations.

Humor Rather Than Snipe

My husband is often frustrated that I suck at hanging towels up to dry. I tend to leave them sitting in the sink. I'm trying to be better at that but I had years of living alone and not sharing that bathroom with anyone. And it doesn't bother *me*. I'm probably gonna use that towel to mop up the floor before I throw it in the laundry, anyway. (Which also grosses him out, but that's another story.)

If I forget to hang up the towel, he will tease me into remembering rather than yell. "Who *hates* to hang up towels?" And I'll wave my hand in the air and say "Me! *Meeee*!" It's obnoxiously cute, but it is way preferable to a stupid fight over a stupid thing, right? I remember to go hang up the towel and neither one of us feel irritated in the process.

Now, someone else having this same conversation might mean it in a mean, snarky, or demeaning way. He's being silly about it, and I take it in kind. The important point is that you find a way to communicate without the sniping, and finding avenues that rely on your shared sense of humor can really help. I've been working with a couple on communicating better with "I" statements. I made a joke about how "I feel you're an asshole" is *not* an I statement. That cracked them up so much that, *"Well, I feel that you're being an asshole"* has become their in-joke that defuses tense conversations.

Beware the Horsemen

Relationship researcher John Gottman is famous for saying he can predict divorce with 90% accuracy. All his research led him to develop what he terms "The Four Horsemen of the Apocalypse." Of his four horsemen, he has found one to be more destructive than all the others. Along with *criticism*, *defensiveness*, and *stonewalling*, the biggest relationship destroyer is the horseman of *contempt*. Contemptuous language—communication that demonstrates you don't respect your partner -- not only becomes a pattern of negative dialogue between the two of you, it reinforces you in thinking about and seeing the negative in your partner.

Gottman also says that the 90% accuracy rate is predicated on people not changing. If you notice that what you are feeling is not just frustration with your partner's choices, but an actual disgust with them as a human being, ask yourself if this is something that you can change with a shift in perspective. If not, you have a pretty good idea about the path you are on.

Ask For What You Need and Negotiate on Things That Are Straight Up Preferences

Communicate your needs (the areas around which you have rigid boundaries) and ask your partner about theirs. If you can't honor these needs in each other and don't think that you would ever be able to, time to abort mission. If someone's need for safety outweighs your capacity to give, that is neither your fault nor theirs. Maybe they have a trauma history that needs more work before they can regain equilibrium. It just is what it is. And like everything else about the human experience, our needs may change over time. Admit when yours change and ask for a renegotiation. Be vulnerable enough to ask for support.

And then there are wants. We all have our preferences and idiosyncrasies. Most of them aren't worth fighting about. Being our own weird, individual selves doesn't mean we are intentionally fucking with our mate, it just means we have years of behavior patterns that are really hard to change. Ever try to give up tacos for Lent? You feel me, right?

Mr. Dr. Faith and I are pains-in-the-asses in a million different ways, but battle stations are only activated when there is a cost involved beyond irritation. I have a toilet paper roll holder that hangs over the side of the toilet tank. Mr. Dr. Faith hates the thing because he has to twist around to reach the roll. He prefers to have the roll to sitting on the counter next to the toilet (*what kind of monster does that???*). I don't like that because it gets damp there. Guess what? We have two rolls of toilet paper in the bathroom. One sitting on the counter and one hanging on the holder. Boom.

What tend to be your relational sticking points? For a lot of people, it's how money is spent. That may mean having an agreement on "allowances"—coming up with an amount that each can spend without checking in with the other based on what you can afford and your financial goals as a couple. Sex troubles? Try out some of the sensate focus exercises in this book to rebuild physical connection. Parenting teenagers? Ugh, good luck with that one.

No matter how big or small, look at the actual cost of the issue before you decide how to proceed. It's amazing how much can be let go when you do that.

Is it Netflix and chill night and you want pizza but boo wants Chinese? Just get both.

Honestly? My goal in life is to have my house be a peaceful abode. I want it to be my favorite place in the world to be. My spouse feels the same, so we work hard at setting up our relationship so we maintain that peace. It's a good goal for all of us.

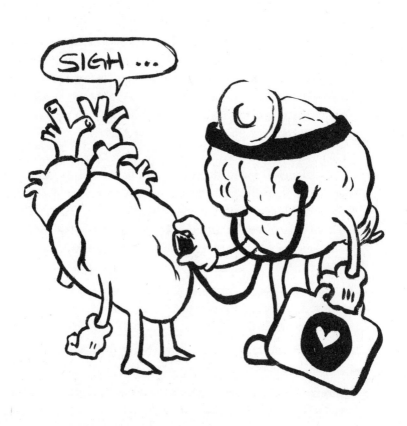

Cheating

P eople cheat. What do I mean by cheating? Anything that doesn't pass the *relationship phone test*. This test is simple as fuck, and I use it with clients on the regular. If your partner were to pick up your phone and opened any of your apps, would they see pictures, posts, or conversations that are in violation of what your relationship rules look like? If so, it's time to do some soul searching.

The relationship phone test is also a great way of checking in on whether or not you are headed into dangerous territory, even if you have convinced yourself that it's not cheating because nothing physical has happened. Remember that each relationship is its own entity and what's okay in one relationship may be a total no-fly in another. Yes, you can be polyamorous and still cheat, if you break relationship rules when engaging with others.

Rates of infidelity vary widely, and research does demonstrate that men cheat more than women. About 40% of men and 25% of women report having violated an agreement of monogamy with a partner overall…and that difference is more pronounced in same-gender relationships, where only 28% of women but 82% of men report having cheated.

As irritating as it is for a feminist to admit, there *are* differences on a global scale between men's and women's levels of sexual desire. It's related to testosterone production. Men think about sex more, want sex more, use porn more, and masturbate more. While

I haven't set seen any research, many transmale and transmasc people have told me anecdotally that starting T revved up their sex drive substantially. If the desire for something is higher, so is the likelihood of engaging in that desire. That doesn't let us women off the hook, though. When we cheat it is more likely to be an affair with a lot of emotional depth, which is far more difficult to recover from.

You may have picked up this book specifically for this chapter. A lot of the people I see in my practice end up there because of infidelity in their relationship. And they are now trying to figure out if the relationship is should and/or can be repaired.

As a therapist, I treat infidelity as a form of interpersonal trauma to the partner who was cheated on. (All good therapists steal from other therapists and my approach to working with infidelity was influenced by the trauma-informed work of Barry McCarthy who was in turn influenced by Snyder, Baucom, and Gordon. References in the back of the book if you're interested.) I am first and foremost a trauma therapist, so this approach makes intuitive sense to me. But I also take a step further, and presume the event was also traumatic to the partner who cheated.

I know I may have lost some of y'all there. Yes, I realize some people are just shitty human beings who have no regard for the feelings of others and no remorse for their behavior. They are just mad as fuck for getting busted and aren't going to do any relationship repair work. If that's the case in your relationship, the hard truth is that you don't really have a relationship based on respect for your needs and value. You've been handed an ultimatum and you need to decide whether or not it's one you can live with.

For everyone else? Yes, the person who was cheated on is clearly, unequivocally injured by what happened. But so was the person who cheated. They did something that was out of alignment to commitments they made and their personal ethical code. It's a form of moral injury that also requires attention and work. When working one-on-one with individuals in affair recovery, I have more clients who cheated than who were cheated on. This includes people who were no longer with the partner they cheated on, because they wanted to figure out what had happened and they didn't want to ever do that again. If they couldn't repair that partnership, they were determined to never hurt anyone else in the same way. I can't even begin to say how impressed I am with the level of emotional maturity that takes.

The good news? Research demonstrates that most relationships *do* recover from an affair. The original school of therapeutic thought was that cheating doomed everything and it was time to just go into Divorce Doula mode with the unhappy couple. Nothing is further from the truth. People fuck up, but if both parties are willing to do the work, the relationship isn't necessarily irreparable. But there are definitely certain things that will greatly increase your chances of surviving, repairing, and being stronger going forward.

Deal With the Emotional Upheaval

When everything first comes out about cheating, shit is intensely volatile. It's helpful to not try to make big decisions during this time period. It's okay to grieve and focus on self-care until you both feel you can commit to communicating with each other more effectively (with or without a therapist present). This may mean taking a break from each other. It definitely means no screaming ragequits and text message fighting. I promise you I have never seen *anything* accomplished by anyone engaged in those types of communication. Going back to your own self-compassion work in the process can be of great benefit for feeling what you are feeling without becoming overwhelmed in the process.

Don't Open Wounds Unnecessarily

You need to focus on what caused the affair to happen and what will prevent it from happening in the future. I have seen lots of people become very wrapped up in needing to know all kinds of details about the affair. And I get the impulse. I really, really do. The person who was cheated on wants to feel back in control of the situation and knowing all the details seems to give a sense of that and feels like it will help them decide if they want to repair the relationship or split up.

I'm not the decider, so I'm not going to stop you. But just like with getting stuck in a volatile emotional state, I've never seen anyone benefit from going through all the minutiae of the affair. It generally only serves to re-wound them over and over again. Remember that you can't unhear information that you ask for. So you need to decide if this information is truly part of your decision making process.

If you are the person who had the affair, withholding the details that are being demanded won't work out well for you in the end. The presumption will be that there are more things you are not telling them, and suspicions will increase. I would try having a conversation about *why* all the details are important (this is a good time to seek professional help, BTW). Should you end up sharing all the details, be prepared to discuss the emotions that are activated.

Get the Information You Need

What kind of information about the affair might be integral to your decision-making process? Some questions that bear consideration for both the cheater and the cheated-on include:

- Is there some evidence that the affair was an escape hatch activity? That is, is there any indication that the cheating partner was looking for the relationship eject button and decided this would do the trick?

- Was the affair with someone of a different gender than that of the partner who was cheated on? That is, is there a question about the cheating partner's sexual orientation that needs to be explored?

- Has the affair ended? Is there any contact with the person with whom the cheating partner had the affair? If so, how is that being managed?

- Were drugs, alcohol, or anything else that induces an altered state of consciousness involved?

- Were barrier protection methods used to minimize the risk for sexually transmitted infections?

- Was the affair an ongoing relationship or a more limited interaction?

- Was the affair sought out in a considered way or did it happen based on opportunity?

- Did the affair contain (or even solely consist of) emotional content? That is, was it just sex or was it also a relationship? Yes, emotional affairs exist. Would the relationship with the other person fail the phone test?

That isn't to say that specific answers equate with "break up" or "stay." I wish it were that easy, but it's definitely not. And I don't need to tell you how something that seems like it should be a clear cut decision is actually one of the hardest decisions you will ever make, no matter what you decide in the end. The point of these questions is to give everyone involved an idea of what you are working with, without getting stuck in the quicksand of the minutiae.

If you and your partner decide to move forward, unpacking the impetus of the affair will be instrumental in reducing the risk of affair relapse. I have found over and over that something was going on either with the person having the affair or within the relationship itself which led them to look for something to make them feel better. Usually what they want is not even sex, but attention, someone to listen to them, or someone to make them feel special and important. But when you start heading down that road, the risk is that you end up slipping and falling into a puddle of sex. And it happens over and over again. Repair is best based on strengthening the original relationship and learning to communicate through disconnection.

Genuinely Own the Cause of the Affair

This means the partner who had the affair needs to take responsibility for their actions, understand what drove these behaviors, request forgiveness genuinely from the partner they cheated on, and commit to doing the work to re-secure their bond and prevent further episodes of cheating.

And this also means the partner who was cheated on has to *believe them*. The apology has to be accepted and trusted as sincere, and the partner who was cheated on has to be equally committed to strengthening the relationship and reconnecting to the person who hurt them. The affair has to stop being defined as the central element of the relationship but seen a consequence of disconnection. This means working on the relationship in the present and planning for the future. It means bringing back basics like date nights. And it means doing things to rebuild emotional and physical intimacy, which may feel awkward and difficult after everything that happened.

Without this commitment by both parties, the chances of authentic relationship repair are pretty fucking slim. I mean, you might stay together while you continue to harbor deep rage, shame, guilt, fear, and pain. But that's not relationship repair. Bravery and vulnerability require commitment and strength from everyone involved.

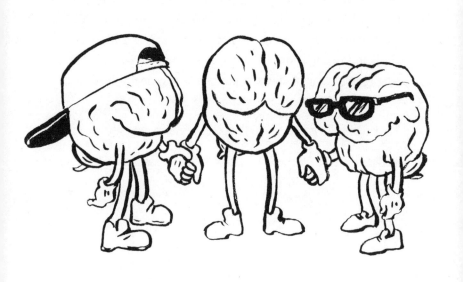

Open Relationships

O pen relationships are greatly misunderstood by most people and nearly all media. There are some great books out there regarding polyamory (check out my recommended reading section for some of them). My intent here is not to reinvent the wheel, but to provide some solid science-y info about open relationships and to point out that not every book about building sexual intimacy is presuming monogamy. Which is why, you will notice, all my advice throughout this book has been polyam inclusive, too.

It's also important to present polyamory within the context of the other things we are talking about. The importance of consent and boundaries. What is and what isn't considered infidelity. Or just the simple fact that being polyam is another valid identity and way of being in the world. So if you are interested in the idea of polyamory, or just want to understand it better, here is some solid info to get your started.

Monogamy: The practice or habit of having one romantic and/or sexual relationship at a time.

Polyamory: The practice or state of being engaged in or open to the idea of having more than one romantic and/or sexual relationship at a time.

Yes, these are very general terms. That's intentional. Many people use the term polyamory to specifically mean relationships, and don't include individuals who are partnered but engage in non-relationship-based sexual exploits like orgies or swinging. However, like Dossie Easton and Janet Hardy (authors of *The Ethical Slut*), I use the term polyamory as an umbrella term for any relationships that are not monogamous, no matter what form they take.

Monogamy is actually pretty rare throughout the animal kingdom, especially among primates. Only 30% of primates are down for monogamy, and only 3% of mammals. Humans are a unique species in that we are wired for both monogamy and polyamory. It's a pretty much straight up 50/50 split. Half of all people prefer monogamy. So you math nerds are already with me on this: the other half dig multiple partners. This holds true of all genders. So the idea that men wanna play and women wanna stay home and raise babies with one mate doesn't hold water.

Our cultural system supports monogamy, as do most secular and spiritual moral codes. But our wiring predates all of these things. So while monogamy is what often makes our social system work, only about half of us are wired for it. And while it seems that *everyone* is in a monogamous relationship, research shows that only 80 to 85% of us actually are.

Hmmmm, right?

A lot of people wired for monogamy are happily monogamous. And yaaay, if you are one of them. Then there are a lot of people who are polyamorous and have slipped through the social norms and created the relationships that work for them. And things are bopping along just fine. (Lots and *lots* of bopping if you are doing things right!) And there are plenty of people in the middle that just aren't sure. The research does show that while 50% of us are wired for polyamory, only about 15-20% of us are practicing some form of it in our current relationship. So there are plenty of people who are maybe interested in polyamory but aren't sure they can make it work…and yeah, it can be difficult.

We have a *lot* of stigma attached to polyamorous relationships. None of the many polyamorous relationships out there have ended up ruining the fabric of society, but the idea still makes many people super uncomfortable. Different usually does. I am always surprised by the number of people who are huge advocates of marriage equality and LGBT rights but are dead set against polyamory as a viable relationship configuration. Other people's relationships are not a threat to yours or to the social structure, no matter how much it may weird you out. I promise.

If your sweetie wants to swing because he found out your neighbors do? Your sweetie was always interested in swinging. The polyam couple down the block didn't turn your sweetie any more than your gay neighbors suddenly made all the straight guys on the street drop their BBQ tongs and weed whackers, trade their Dockers for assless chaps, and develop a hankering to go to disco night at Wild Zebra.

All that being said, what if polyamory *is* your problem? Or interest? Or hmmmmmm moment? Or you found a pair of assless chaps in the back of your sweetie's closet? How is all that supposed to work?

CCR, baby: Consent, Communication, and Respect.

These are things that should happen in every relationship but are *absolutely* the keys to the successful polyamorous relationships that I have seen. And some of the healthiest relationships I have seen are polyamorous in some form or another. Yes, seriously.

What does this mean in practical terms if you are considering this? Awesome question!

Dr. Faith's Rules for Navigating Polyamory

1. Polyamory doesn't exist only in one partner's mind. It is negotiated adultery, for lack of a better term. I shouldn't have to say this part but I have had to say it and apparently continue to need to say it: If your partner doesn't know about your side activities, you are not polyamorous, you're cheating. Don't be a dick.

2. If you have a relationship fraught with all kinds of problems, and polyamory is your last-ditch effort to stay together? You won't. You will only prolong your breakup, make it messier, and create more heartache. Just break up.

3. Be open but don't be pushed. This means if you have a partner who is asking you to consider polyamory, be willing to actually consider it. But you don't have to be pushed or pressured or do anything that you absolutely don't want to do. If this is something you and your partner are exploring, look at all the different ways your relationship can be opened up and see if any are in your comfort zone. Also consider different ways you can spice up your relationship while remaining monogamous. Sometimes we need something different and we don't know what different is. Look at options before trying anything. There are plenty of meet and greet groups where you can explore without being action-oriented. Check out Meetup or FetLife scheduled events, or just do a google search for polyamory + [area you live in] to find your local folx.

4. Do what's right for you, your partner, and the relationship. The rules vary widely depending on what works for people, from "I want to meet anyone before you sleep with them" to "Don't tell me anything about them, I just know Wednesday nights are your date nights." Some people use polyamory for certain activities that their primary partner isn't in to, while others prefer a fully shared third partner joining their family. What do *you* want it to look like? Something you do together? Something completely separate? Only people you know and trust? Only people you don't know at all? Only people who are clearly not *nearly* as hot as you are? (I kinda like the idea of this one, just sayin'!)

5. Negotiate the *hell* out of your relationship rules (scaffolding, whatever word works) and renegotiate as much as you need to. If you thought something was going to be fine and then you went bat shit crazy jealous? Own that and work through it. Don't seethe quietly in the corner while your partner is thinking everything is okay until you go kaboom one random Sunday afternoon when your partner leaves the toilet seat up. (And yes, I know, in your defense, they do that *all the fucking time and you are over it!*) The authors of *The Ethical Slut* suggest having a plan for when jealousy hits. If you plan how to handle such feelings in a way that reconnects and strengthens the relationship, it's far less likely to reach a breaking point.

6. Depending on the level of involvement of the secondary partner(s), include them in the negotiations. I have worked with primary and secondary partners in therapy, figuring out their issues regarding an individual with whom they both had a relationship. How great is it that they brought everything to the

table and worked together? Sometimes it only took one session of honest convo to get everything back on track.

7. Consider how these choices can affect other areas of your life and how you want to handle this. Whose business is it? Do you tell people? How do you discuss it if they find out? What about if you have kiddos? Have a plan for these inevitabilities so you can act rather than react.

8. Find health care providers who don't shame you for your choices. Make sure your docs know that you engage in activities that mean you need regular STI testing, for example (and, it should also go without saying, but practice safer sex, FFS!), and don't let them give you any shit about your relationships. Its generally easier to find a polyam-friendly therapist than it is a polam friendly MD. Those of us who specialize in intimacy will announce straight out on our Psychology Today profiles and our websites if we are polyam friendly and kink aware. Another place to look is on the site listings for Kink Aware Professionals (KAP) or ask around the local polyam and kink communities.

9. Don't demand that everyone have the same level of involvement and commitment. I've seen couples have healthy polyam relationships where one partner was a hardwired polyamorist and the other wasn't. They were truly okay with it, didn't have a jealous streak, had amazing communication, and wanted their partner to be happy. Some people are generally down for polyam play as a couple but not as invested in dating the way their polyam partner is. This has happened enough times, that I ended up developing a new polyam label in session a couple of years ago: *sushi-polyam*. It comes from the fact that one of my husband's favorite meals is sushi. He seriously digs sushi.

I like sushi just fine. But it's not a hardcore favorite and so it's not on my mental rolodex of menus. If you ask me what I want for dinner I will probably say "tacos" but if you say "sushi sound okay?" I'm likely to say "Sure!" I have zero problem saying no to things I don't want. Sushi is delicious. I just don't crave it. So if you have a sushi-polyam partner, that's OK. They don't have to be as excited about it to be perfectly content with the dynamic. And if they aren't content? They are responsible for themselves and what they agree to. If they are secretly unhappy, it's up to them to divulge that.

10. Because I am a sucker for a list of ten rules, I'm going to throw in one more: Don't let other people determine your self-worth. There are only a handful of people in this world whose opinion of me actually matters to me. The rest of the eleventy billion people on the planet don't get a vote, no matter how much they think they should. Your doctor, your therapist, and anyone else in your life do not get a vote on how you handle your intimate relationships. Only you and the individual(s) you are in these relationships with do. If something isn't right for you or your relationship, then don't do it. But not because Aunt Susie says so. You are allowed to seek the types of relationships that are supportive, invigorating, and fun for you, whether they be monogamous or polyamorous. Consider this a note from your doctor.

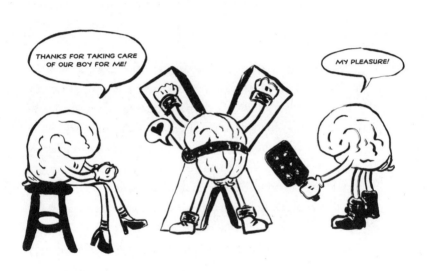

Kinks, Fets, and BDSM (Oh Myyyyyyyyy)

Maybe you want to be blindfolded or maybe you fantasize about being suspended upside down. Maybe you are intrigued by furries. Or love the idea of sex in a wading pool full of Jell-o. Whatever interests you are chatting to yourself about doesn't make you weird. There's a lot of interesting brain science-y stuff about what makes us interested in more interesting sexcapades. And if you fall in this category, it's all really good news. And hey, even if you don't? It's all super interesting... and you may end up with a partner or a buddy that's a kinkster and you want to understand their experience better. It's more common than you'd think!

Fetishes

First, some terminology because there is always overlap and general vagueness in sexual health topics that annoys the shit out of me:

A **kink** is merely the overarching term used to describe sexual behaviors that are considered *unconventional*. Of course, unconventional is based on individual cultural criteria of what "normal" is, so good luck defining it any further than that, right?

A *fetish* is something that becomes psychologically necessary for sexual gratification, either by needing to be present or imagined during sexual activity. If something exists, someone out there has a fetish for it. It could be body parts (women's feet for example), objects, or a specific behavior (like watching others have sex). Interestingly, other than the fets associated with BDSM, fetish behavior is almost exclusively something that men engage in. Which means that there is something about object fetish for stimulation that is somehow linked to testosterone. This is kinda important, because it reinforces that we have biological preferences. Meaning, because I can't say this enough in response to societal messages that state otherwise, that having a fetish doesn't mean that what you are into is a perversion, weirdness, or abuse-driven behavior.

Some fets end up getting people in serious trouble, like voyeurism. In this case, the fet itself isn't the problem, it's lack of consent. If you are watching porn about your fetish or at a venue where it's an agreed-upon activity (there are people out there who like being watched just like there are people who like to watch, after all) then it's all good. Problems happen when people try to fill their fet need but have so much shame around their interest that they end up acting out in public spaces or otherwise around people who are not consenting to the behavior they're engaging in.

Chances are, if you're into kink and fetish stuff, it's because you are a naturally hypersexual person. Research demonstrates that people of all genders who are hypersexual are the ones that are most likely to be into non-vanilla sex. *Hypersexual* is a bit of a loaded word, and that is such bullshit. It tends to be used to label someone as sexually dysfunctional, but really just means they have more sex than 95% of the population. And no matter what sex shamers say, liking and having lots of sex is not dysfunctional. Let's be honest *"too much sex"* is usually defined by people as *"more sex than I have"* as if that's a standard unit of measure. If you're into it? *Treat. Yo. Self.*

The correlation between being hypersexual and having more varied interests makes sense, right? If you are into sex and generally have a lot of sex, you are looking for ways to make it fun, and interesting, and stimulating. If you only ate meals a few times a month, getting a hamburger and fries each time wouldn't be a big deal. But if you eat every day, or several times a day, you probably want some variety in your meals, right? I throw this little tidbit in here not just because I'm a research geek, but because I've had sooooo many clients find it helpful to know that their interests are a natural expansion of their sex drive.

And hopefully it's pretty obvious that it doesn't mean that the non-hypersexual people with kink and fet interests are weird and aberrant. No stats in this regard, but my clinical experience tells me that we are all wired to like what we like. And people who have kinks and fets often had interests in these things even as very young children, way before puberty. Meaning they found something intriguing and when they become sexually active adolescents and adults, that became a natural place to express that interest.

Entire books about specific kinks and fetishes are out there, so going into great detail about all or any of them is quite impossible. But because BDSM is the most prevalent form of kink/fet sexual intimacy, and because mainstream media often portrays it so very badly, it does bear some extra consideration here.

BDSM

BDSM (also sometimes referred to as S&M) stands for Bondage / Domination / Sadism / Masochism. Depending on who you talk to, the D may stand for discipline instead of domination and the S may stand for submission instead of sadism. Either way, it's a catchall term for erotic control play, and it is nothing like the way the *Fifty Shades* books and movies presented it to be.

Let's go a little bit beyond the literal definition.

BDSM has what we call the "Three Cs": Consent, Control, and Communication.

Consent: BDSM is always based on consent for all parties involved. Consent fluctuates and can change and adapt over time. Consent is negotiated ahead of time and negotiated through the interaction.

Control: BDSM is about control in many different forms, not just the control of one human being by another. The dom also has to be in complete control of themself at all times in order to respect the boundaries and ensure the safety of their sub.

Communication: BDSM is seriously, seriously, seriously about communication. You have to talk about everything going on before, during, and after the experience. You may consent to something and realize later you hit a boundary you didn't realize existed. Your interests may change and fluctuate over encounters or periods of time. What makes BDSM healthy is the fact that involved parties are constantly having conversations about what is going on.

There are a ton of studies out there. 10-25% of people in most studies report being turned on by aspects of BDSM, about 2-25% have actually tried BDSM in the past year (depends on how well the study defines BDSM!). The vast majority of people have said they have definitely fantasized about it. So there you go, you aren't nearly alone.

Another seriously important (and pretty cool) research point? People who are involved in BDSM tend to be *more* emotionally healthy than the rest of us. When studying different personality traits, BDSM practitioners reported higher levels of well-being, were more open to new experiences in general and were more extraverted, less rejection-sensitive, more conscientious, and less neurotic than the general population.

Research shows the one less desirable personality trait BDSM practitioners possess is that they are less agreeable. Which cracks me up because I take this to mean that BDSM practitioners are better at standing up for themselves and not doing things they aren't comfortable with. Yeah, not so much a negative.

BDSM is usually about sex, but not always. Sometimes BDSM is about the mindfuck rather than the act of sex. It's a turn-on, but no erogenous stimulation is taking place. You may have noticed in the initial definition of BDSM that it's about the arousal and growth more than physical release.

Pain may not be involved at all, either. It's about power and control. There are many levels to this. It may be a matter of the dominant partner directing all the actions of the submissive one. It may include being tied up with scarves and tickled with a feather. It may mean spankings. It may mean hardcore needle play. YMMV. And *it's your choice.*

BDSM exists on a continuum. Kinda like going to the gym. Some people go every day and have serious rock hard abs. Some go a couple times a week and do a little cardio. Some people only get exercise when reaching for the box of cookies. You can do super-pervy with extra kinky sauce or a little vanilla with sprinkles.

Of course the more you play, the more careful you have to be because the more risk (emotional and physical) is involved. You stay safe by minimizing the risks and learning what you are doing before you start. And you always have an escape hatch, like a safe word. Reading and talking to others in the community is extremely beneficial for safety if you plan to go beyond anything very basic.

For example, if your interest is tying up, you don't want to knot the rope (or scarves, or whatever you are using), since a knot can easily cut off circulation and be difficult to untie in a hurry. There are resources to help you learn tying techniques that protect your sub partner. While tied up, you need to be able to maintain constant communication about your ability to maintain circulation. If you struggle to notice circulation issues in yourself (for example, you are diabetic and have neuropathy), your dom partner may ask you to push up against their hand to show that you aren't numb, and they need to have an implement available to immediately cut you free if needed.

Being a submissive in a BDSM relationship does not mean you are giving up all control. In fact, it is the polar opposite. The sub in a BDSM relationship is the one with all the power. The dom has to be in complete control of themselves in order to ensure that boundaries are not crossed, that their sub is always safe, and that they can immediately stop if the safe word is utilized. That is a lot of power and the sub has most of it. This can be a powerfully healing experience for some people with trauma backgrounds. If you are an abuse survivor, the main question to ask yourself about your BDSM relationship is: Do you feel secure and in control of the experience or not? If the answer is no or not sure, seeing a trauma-trained therapist to help you figure some of that out might make a lot of sense.

No matter what your background, each BDSM interaction should include "straight time" at the end to discuss the experience. Some people even set up contracts for their playtime, which can provide legal safety and make everyone involved feel more secure, especially if this is a new thing for you.

Don't freak out though—BDSM can be experimental and light fun. Not everything has to involve a drama llama of a contract. BDSM is like an onion. Lots of layers. Hopefully, none of them make you cry, though. Unless, of course, that's your thing.

Fantasy and Role-Play

A fantasy is a mental image, not necessarily something you act on. Role-play, on the other hand, means acting or performing a role or character that is somewhat different from your day to day life.

While BDSM can definitely have a fantasy and role-play component (and yes, you could argue that all BDSM is a form of role-play), you can also engage in fantasy and role-play without having the power differential component of BDSM.

To be honest, I hadn't really thought about role-play being its own separate entity until a number of my gender non-conforming clients talked about their use of it in sexual intimacy. If people trust me enough to talk about that stuff, I totally need to listen. And I found that, as with BDSM, the experience can be profoundly healing when approached in the right way. So let's address a few points.

Fantasy Doesn't Mean Reality

The checklist I use with clients about sexual activities has four options: yes, no, I don't know, and fantasy only. Being intrigued by an idea or turned on by it isn't the same thing as being interested in trying it out in real life.

About 75% of our sexual fantasies are about sexual activities that we have engaged in or intend to engage in. Whatever our definition of "normal" sex may be. Which means the other 25% are about things that have some level of intrigue for us but aren't something we necessarily want to try out.

When studying both heterosexual and homosexual men, Masters and Johnson Institute researchers found that both groups fantasized about having sex with a person not of their traditional orientation. That was as high on the list as BDSM fantasies, group sex fantasies, and all of the other common fantasies that people experience.

A 2015 study found that that up to 62% of women in the study had experienced rape fantasies. Do 62% of women secretly harbor a desire to be raped? Maybe some losers on 4chan think so, but I seriously doubt it. The researcher looked at how often the fantasy occurred, and it wasn't often. Once a week, maybe once a month. And it wasn't tied to the idea of not having to take responsibility for a sexual encounter but was actually tied to younger generations (millennials and Zers) being experientially open and fantasy allowing them to express that without actual violation.

So much of what we fantasize about does not reflect our true interests. I've had clients tell me with great horror how they told their partner about a fantasy they had. But when their partner went to the trouble of trying to fulfill it for them, my clients were embarrassed to find that they actually had no real interest.

You may have seen articles that decry the porn industry as depicting too much violence, specifically violence towards women. Interestingly, the studies that set out to quantify violence in porn range substantially (2% to 88% percent…HUGE difference!). Mostly because we all define violence differently. For instance, is consensual BDSM considered violence? I wouldn't say so, but others may (she says while rolling her eyes).

Finding yourself drawn to some level of physical force doesn't make you a violent person, nor does it mean you are going to go out and act violently toward others. Brain science time: Sex and violence responses are essentially one and the same. Both activities involve stimulation of a specific part of the brain (the ventral medial hypothalamus). The only difference is in the *level* of the neuron activity: there is more activity during episodes of violence than during sex. So if you are an otherwise chill person who uses porn or has fantasies that involves a show of physical force, that may just be your brain amping up your neuron activity in that region for purposes of sexual excitement. You aren't automatically qualified as having a problem, okay?

Fantasy allows us to explore other ways of being in the world, expressing ourselves, and "trying things on for size." Our brains are wired for storytelling, and fantasy is just storytelling. It's how we process our perceptions and experience possibilities. If your fantasies distress you or you find yourself wanting to act on certain things that are harmful, hurtful, or illegal, *that's* the time to seek help. Fantasies alone are a normal human experience.

Role-Play

In my practice, I've seen a huge jump in clients who are into sexual role-play. As a Gen Xer, I definitely knew about furry parties and the like, but the internet has made it so much easier to find people with similar interests and engage in sex with them, setting up elaborate stories and settings in which we can enact certain roles that would be otherwise impossible or inappropriate. The obvious example is the dude who wants to relive his high school glory days by having his partner wear a cheerleading uniform. That's not the same as them trying to hook up with a 14-year-old cheerleader, right? Or maybe you are into firefighters but you are in a monogamous relationship with someone who isn't a firefighter. Maybe they are willing to put on the suit and come put out your metaphorical fire for you.

Role-play (within BDSM or otherwise) can also be a safe place to explore your rougher fantasies (the stuff that falls under the heading of "violent" for lack of a better term). If that's the kind of thing that gets you going, role-play can allow you to have that experience within the boundaries of safeties and limits intended to protect you from unwanted harm.

I've also seen roleplay be beneficial and healing for my clients who are trans or otherwise gender non-conforming. If you feel uncomfortable with your physical body presentation, role-playing as someone else allows you a new level of freedom. Many younger clients told me that non-sexual role-playing games brought their first self-awareness of their gender identity and that starting in puberty they found themselves picking characters of their authentic gender instead of birth assignment.

And it should be noted that a lot of people are just big fans of certain characters and really enjoy cosplay. Bringing that cosplay into their sexual relationships simply enhances the experience. You don't need to hate your body in order to enjoy being someone else now and then!

Things to Watch Out For

While I am totally the queen of *"you do you and let your freak flag fly,"* sexual fantasy and role-play can end up being problematic. Just like anything else fun, right? Here are some warning signs:

1) Just like with sex and porn misuage, if the fantasy and role-play take the place of real engagement with other human beings there might be a problem

2) If your fantasies do move into perseveration territory, meaning they occupy your thoughts and you feel impulses to act on things you know are wrong or find disturbing

3) If your partners are violating your boundaries under the guise of the role-play, including online, it isn't real sex. It's important to set and keep boundaries (in character or out) that protect you from being hurt. (Tip from a gamer friend: Announce that you are having connection issues and log out if you don't want to have a conversation about why you're leaving.)

If you are noticing patterns of problem behavior in yourself, find a sex-positive, kink-aware professional (therapist, body worker) to work with on developing better usage strategies and coping skills.

Differential Desires

Sometimes your partner (or whomever you are having sex with) wants something different, sexually, than you do. There doesn't seem to be any rhyme or reason to whether or not this person lets you know right away or after decades of being together. Sometimes, and usually with ungreat timing, boo drops a bombshell on you.

It could be anything from the kink, fet, and BDSM menu. It could be something utterly different like maybe they are ace, or poly, or any of the many other ways people can be in the world. Since I've been dropping some science throughout this book about all of these topics, you're with me on the fact that these are all very normal ways of being in the world.

So what do you do with that? You can part ways, totally. Consciously uncouple Gwyneth Paltrow style, sure. Or maybe there is some room for negotiation? Here are some ideas.

Negotiate Your Boundaries

Maybe your partner is the one who wants to role-play their fantasy, and you now realize that doesn't mean they have a fucked-up, psychopathic dark side but it's still something you are not OK with? Do not do a *damn* thing you don't want to do. This is not *Fifty Shades of Grey*, where someone is going to push you past your comfort zone without permission. Because even pushing you out of your comfort zone requires consent. No consent, no play.

But if it doesn't freak you out, and does lovely things for them? That's what partnership is all about, right? Boo is into diaper play? Maybe the rule will be, "Fine, I'm good with the diaper, but if you crap the thing you are on your own." Boo wants to gag you? Ok, bandana is fine, but if a ball gag shows up in the bedroom, boo gets a nut-punch. I dated a guy who was into feet. *Really* into feet. Feet don't do anything for me but it made him happy and I got a free pedicure out of the deal. Negotiation.

Most importantly, boundaries are not written in stone. They can be renegotiated all the time. If you both don't feel safe in having those conversations, then it really won't work. There can't be any, "Well, last week you said…" Consent, consent, consent. And that is as fluid as sexuality.

Consider a Pinch Hitter

Many polyamorous relationships are based on fulfilling differential desires. The thing about polyamory is, again, consent. Everyone is on the same page, everyone knows what the rules are, and everyone knows what the limits are.

Differential desires don't mean you have to dump the baby out with the bathwater. Say boo is into needle play. You are in *no way* into needle play. So the deal is, you go to a local club and boo gets to engage in the needle play. You can go and watch. Or you can stay home and play Cards Against Humanity with your friends. Whatever. Boo is allowed to play with predetermined limits and you are needle-free. Or maybe boo is polyam and you aren't, so you go to the swingers club together to watch the action without participating. Maybe you involve porn or fantasy-talk about their polyam interests in your sex life to get them revved up without opening the relationship. Maybe Boo like prostate stimulation and you are uncomfortable with being the stimulator so they use a toy for that while y'all are doing other sexitimes stuff together. I'm just sayin'...we got options here.

Figure out what you think you will be comfortable with, make a plan, and make another plan to manage any issues that may arise. The upshot is that differential desires don't have to be a deal-breaker. All relationships are a dance. Fred Astaire did just fine with a coat rack, but most of us prefer an actual partner in that dance. And if you have an excellent boo who always does the dishes when you do the cooking, there is no harm in trying to work it out.

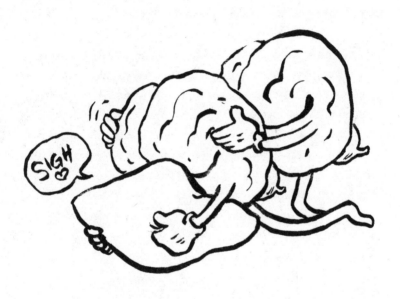

Sensate Touch

Sensate touch exercises (also called sensate focus exercises) were developed by Masters and Johnson to help couples work through intimacy issues. They are included in this book as the final chapter because they are very helpful in rebuilding partner intimacy regardless of what caused the problem to begin with. I consider sensate focus exercises another relationship skill, just like date night, effective communication, and all the other shit I yammer on about.

In Part One I talked about the levels of touch: healing, sensual, erotic, and sexual. All forms of touch are important in our romantic partnerships and all help foster a sense of intimacy, and these exercises were designed to build on all four of these levels. One of the most important ways of doing that is not only improving our communication about touch, but also finding true enjoyment in both giving and receiving touch from our partners.

One of the biggest barriers to fostering intimate touch, both sexual and non-sexual, is the expectation of return demonstration. Instead, the giver should focus on the pleasure experienced in touching their partner, rather than focusing on what they get when it is "their turn." All relationships have a give and take, but except for the first pre-touch exercise here, time always should be set aside for the receiver to enjoy the experience without being expected to return the favor. Giving pleasure for its own sake to your partner can be its own intensely rewarding experience that fosters intimacy in and of itself.

There are many variations of these exercises out there. I designed my version to be both trauma-mindful and trauma-informed. But these exercises can be modified for *any* reason you need, okay?

Goals of the Exercises

- To learn how we like to be touched.

- To learn how our partner likes to be touched.

- To find new ways to explore our needs and desires.

- To find new ways of receiving and giving pleasure without focusing on immediate sexual release.

- To demonstrate to ourselves and our partner a commitment to our relationship.

- To help build connection and deepen our relationship with our partner.

- To become more comfortable with our physical selves as our bodies evolve and change through childbirth, aging, and/or disability.

Establish Ground Rules

Before you begin, it's a good idea to discuss what you hope to accomplish. It's a good idea to establish some boundaries up front:

- Determine if there are any areas that you do not want to have touched, and how you will communicate if that changes during the exercises. Consider a safe word or gesture if you are concerned that you may struggle with communicating your needs.

- Decide ahead of time if you desire to be clothed, partially clothed, or naked during the earlier stage sensate touch exercises.

- Consider how you will handle any unexpected outcomes. For example, one partner or both may become sexually aroused and want to engage in more than sensate touch. There is no rule, of course, that you cannot engage in activities other than sensate touch during your touch sessions, however neither partner should feel pressured to do so. Having a plan on how to handle those issues ahead of time will help prevent hurt feelings or unfulfilled expectations.

Afterwards, talk about your experiences and whether or not you think the goals you set at the beginning are being achieved. Discuss the positives and negatives of each encounter. Use "I" statements to demonstrate your own accountability for your thoughts and feelings.

How to Do the Exercises

Once you've talked over your goals and boundaries, pick a time and place where you will feel comfortable and won't be interrupted by other people or by the telephone, TV, or other intrusions. For the sensate focus exercises, consider doing them in the morning if a male partner is the receiver, as testosterone levels are highest in the morning. Use lighting that feels comfortable to you and music if you find that soothing. If you aren't using your bed for the initial exercises (which makes sense if that's become a source of pressure), you can still use plenty of pillows and blankets to feel comfortable wherever you are.

Use lotions, oils, or a powder for the massage exercises (make sure to use one that is face friendly for the face caress, like a moisturizing cream). Some people find lotions and oils to be slimy and prefer talc or cornstarch (which doesn't clump, is cheap AF, and is probably already in your pantry). For the exercises that include genital stimulation, you may want to use a lubricant. This can be especially helpful if a female partner has issues producing enough lubrication due to menopause or other medical conditions or if a male partner struggles to maintain a full erection. If you have not used lubricant before, read all the labels and test it out on a small area on your skin to make sure you do not have an allergic reaction. Remember not to use oil-based lubrication when using condoms or silicone-based lubricants when using silicone-based toys.

Alternate being the giver and the receiver. You can take turns during the same occasion or set separate times so the receiver can fully enjoy the experience, without having to return the favor after they are relaxed.

The person receiving the touch should state what feels good and what does not. Communicate this using "I" statements. "I like it when…" and "I don't like…" rather than "You shouldn't…" or "Stop that!" Positive redirection such as "I prefer…" always feels best to the giving partner. Positive feedback in general is always preferred, especially noises of appreciation when your partner does something you especially enjoy!

The giver should ask for feedback about areas of touch, pressure, and technique. One way to learn what the receiver likes is letting them guide your hand, especially at first. Consider using your non-dominant hand for times when a lighter touch is preferred. As you notice your partner's response to receiving certain types of stimulation, take time to focus on the sensations you feel as the giver. What does your partner's skin feel like? What does the part of your body touching them feel like as you move over their skin?

There is no time limit or limit to the number of sessions you spend on any exercise or stage. You can spend as much time as you want on each exercise before moving to the next one in order to establish comfort and trust. It is important that partners do not pressure each other to move forward until both are ready to do so. It can be very helpful to spend several weeks on a particular stage and exercise, incorporating a bit more of the body or areas of the body each time you practice.

Remember, the aim of these exercises is enjoyment, relaxation, connectedness, and pleasure. Focus on the journey rather than the end result.

Pre-Touch Shared Breathing Exercise

Sit facing each other. Maintaining eye contact, slow your breathing and focus on breathing in unison. If you don't have medical issues that disrupt your breathing patterns, try to breathe in to the count of three, hold for the count of three, and release your breath for a count of three. Focus your thoughts on loving intent toward your partner, such as "I choose you" or "I care for you."

Continue this pattern for two minutes. Two minutes will seem like a very long time the first time you try this! You can continue these exercises over time, extending the amount of time you spend in shared breathing.

Discuss the experience with your partner. What did you notice? Did anything make you uncomfortable? Was there anything you particularly enjoyed?

The Hand Caress

Sit in a comfortable position, facing each other. Using a lotion, oil, or powder gently rub your partner's hand. Spend 5-10 minutes on each hand (10-20 minutes total). Explore each finger, the pads of their fingers, the lines of their palms. Check in with your partner about the amount of pressure you are using. Focus your thoughts on loving intent toward your partner such as "I choose you" or "I care for you."

Discuss the experience with your partner. What did you notice? Did anything make you uncomfortable? Was there anything you particularly enjoyed?

The Face Caress

Pick a position that is most comfortable for you. Many people find it works best if the giver is sitting and the receiver is lying flat on their back with their head resting on the giver's thighs. The giver should first rub a facial-friendly lubricant, like a moisturizing lotion, or powder like corn starch on their hands. Begin with the chin, then stroke the cheeks, temples, and forehead. Check in with your partner about the amount of pressure that you are using. Explore your partner's earlobes, and the indentation just behind the earlobes on the neck. Return to massaging the temples. This exercise should take about 10-20 minutes. Focus your thoughts on loving intent toward your partner such as "I choose you" or "I care for you."

Discuss the experience with your partner. What did you notice? Did anything make you uncomfortable? Was there anything you particularly enjoyed?

Sensate Body Work

You may have noticed that the first exercises were more in the healing and possibly sensual domain. This is where we start to move into erotic and sexual!

Stage One

Limit touching and stroking to areas of the body that are not sexually stimulating. Start with areas that feel safe for your partner and incorporate more areas on future turns. Oftentimes, individuals have the first session lying on their back, being touched only on the front of their body, where they can see everything their partner is doing. If that feels comfortable, start a later session with the receiver laying on their stomach and having you work on their neck, shoulders, back, and backs of arms and legs.

You can continue to include the hands and face, but also include feet, legs, and arms. Be careful for areas that are ticklish. Continue to focus your thoughts on loving intent toward your partner such as "I choose you" or "I care for you."

Discuss the experience with your partner. What did you notice? Did anything make you uncomfortable? Was there anything you particularly enjoyed?

Stage Two

Start with the touch you used in the first stage before moving on. During the second stage, you can include genital areas in the places you touch and stroke, but the intent at this point is not sexual arousal but sensual response.

Often during stage two, individuals find it works best to start by incorporating touch of the breasts and nipples, then touching areas around the genitals. Oral touching as well as manual touching can be introduced here (or in later stages) if both partners are comfortable with it, such as light kissing, licking, or sucking.

Continue to focus your thoughts on loving intent toward your partner such as "I choose you" or "I care for you."

Discuss the experience with your partner. What did you notice? Did anything make you uncomfortable? Was there anything you particularly enjoyed?

Stage Three

Start with the touch you used in the first two stages before moving to the third. During the third stage, include touch of the genitals with intention to arouse. On a woman, stroke the clitoris and/or gently probe the vaginal opening with a finger. On men, stroke the shaft of the penis, and the head of the penis (including the frenulum, which is the spot where the head and the shaft of the penis join). On either partner, this can include stroking the anus if the receiving partner has expressed a desire for you to do so.

Continue to focus your thoughts on loving intent toward your partner such as "I choose you" or "I care for you."

Discuss the experience with your partner. What did you notice? Did anything make you uncomfortable? Was there anything you particularly enjoyed?

Stage Four

Start with the touch you used in the first three stages before moving to the fourth. And, as with the other stages, not doing this one at all is completely fine. If penetrative intercourse, however, is something you want to include in your sex life, stage four is designed to get you there.

During the fourth stage, you can attempt vaginal or anal penetration either with a finger, penis or sexual aid, depending on your partner's preference. The extent of penetration and what you use for penetration and where you experience penetration is entirely up to you. For example, individuals with vaginas who experience vaginismus (an involuntary contraction of the muscles around the opening of the vagina) may need to start with a q-tip or a small vaginal dilator before even a finger is a tenable option.

Continue to focus your thoughts on loving intent toward your partner such as "I choose you" or "I care for you."

Discuss the experience with your partner. What did you notice? Did anything make you uncomfortable? Was there anything you particularly enjoyed?

These are exercises you can continue using or go back to regularly as you find them helpful.

Conclusion

O k, wow. That was a lot. Did you read all the way through? Are you totally exhausted? Hey, I don't blame you.

This book was intended to be full of bite-sized pieces of all the sexual and relational intimacy work I have learned and utilized over the years. It comes from the questions I've asked, and the stuck places I've seen with clients in my practice. It's not all-encompassing and it doesn't replace intensive individual or couples therapy. But hopefully, there were places where you read just the right question to help facilitate an "aha!" moment about your own life. Or you hit upon an interesting resource you had never seen before and you have a new plan of attack about something that has felt pretty overwhelming in the past.

We all deserve a healthy and fulfilling sex life. And we all get to determine what that looks like for us. Fighting for a meaningful and fulfilling life is something we do in other places, right? We vote, we floss, and we even eat broccoli instead of donuts on occasion. And this is no more frivolous work.

My hope is that this book leads to more open discussions about sexual intimacy in general. We don't do this nearly enough. If we did, I might just be out of a job and this book will fall out of print because it had become absolutely unnecessary. And I'd totally be down with that.

The topic of sexual intimacy invokes a lot of overwhelm for most people. All the blame and shame and stigma around our identities as sexual beings is hugely overwhelming. But that doesn't mean we're stuck in that place. It's not easy or intuitive work. Unfucking our intimacy issues requires practical, pragmatic strategies. If you wanted to cook a flan and didn't grow up in a flan-cooking culture you'd have to learn that shit, right? Same with a healthy sex life. That's why this book is full of practical strategies instead of romantic ideals. Because that's what unfuckening requires, right?

Let's get busy.[1]

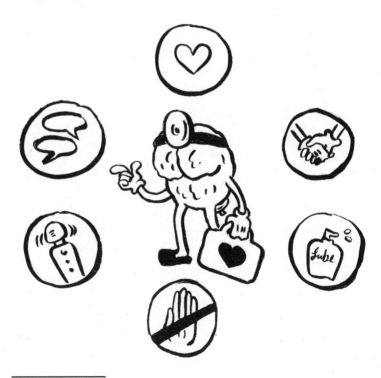

---

1 I mean, if you're consenting. And you're into that kinda thing. Of course.

Further Reading and Resources

Abusive Relationships

If you know (or are starting to suspect) your relationship is abusive, I hope you will consider creating a safety plan for yourself. Cover what to do if you plan to stay, or for when you decide to leave. You do not have to be living with a violent partner to need or have a safety plan. Some safety planning tools I recommend include:

- The Domestic Violence Safety Plan by Kellie Holly (www.verbalabusejournals.com) - this is the most comprehensive plan
- The National Domestic Violence Hotline Safety Planning (www.thehotline.org) - specifically includes help on planning to leave when you have pets
- Scarleteen Safety Plans (available on their website, www.scarleteen.com) - includes a separate plan to use if you don't live with your abuser
- The military has developed a safety plan specific to the needs of having a service-member partner (DD Form 2893)

Affirming, Sex-Positive Sexuality

Sex Outside the Lines: Authentic Sexuality in a Sexually Dysfunctional Culture by Chris Donaghue

Unpacks the bullshit around the stigma of sex and encourages self-discovery and self-acceptance.

Sex From Scratch: Making Your Own Relationship Rules by Sarah Mirk

A love and dating guidebook that gleans real-life knowledge from smart people in a variety of nontraditional relationships.

BDSM, Kink, and Fet

SM 101: A Realistic Introduction by Jay Wiseman

The classic. A great overview of BDSM with good general information on getting started with exploring the lifestyle.

The Ultimate Guide to Kink: BDSM, Role Play and the Erotic Edge by Tristan Taormino

A great series of essays ranging from how-tos to think pieces about exploring power, pleasure, and human desire.

When Someone You Love Is Kinky by Dossie Easton

Very helpful for non-kinky folx who are looking to better understand and communicate with their kinky partners.

Boundaries and Consent

Learning Good Consent: Building Ethical Relationships in a Complicated World by Cindy Crabb

This compilation has fantastic information about applying boundaries and maintaining consent in real-life, sticky situations.

Ask: Building Consent Culture by Kitty Stryker

A guide to creating a culture of consent, and not just in the bedroom.

Consensuality: Navigating feminism, gender, and boundaries towards loving relationships by Helen Wildfell

A guide to creating or finding a healthy, successful relationship as well as avoiding common pitfalls.

Changing Bodies & Disabilities

The Ultimate Guide to Sex and Disability: For All of Us Who Live with Disabilities, Chronic Pain, and Illness by Miriam Kaufman, Cory Silverberg, and Fran Odette

Covers the multitude of ways disability can create obstacles to a healthy sex life along with great tips for overcoming these obstacles.

Guide To Getting It On by Paul Joannides

Recent editions of the print book have been abridged, so the chapter on sex and disability is now online for free download. Woot! But, FWIW, the book itself has great info in general.

Sexual Intelligence by Marty Klein

About communication and pragmatic expectations and the emotional work it takes to make sexual intimacy good when nobody involved in the relationship is a perfect performer. Not overtly about changing bodies but it actually totally *is* about just this topic.

Fantasies

Who's Been Sleeping in Your Head: The Secret World of Sexual Fantasies by Brett Kahr

The result of one of the largest studies ever done on sexual fantasy, with over 23,000 participants. Amazing information about what our sexual fantasies say about the nature of being human.

Tell Me What You Want: The Science of Sexual Desire and How It Can Help You Improve Your Sex Life by Justin J. Lehmiller

A researcher for The Kinsey Institute (toothbrush guy!!!) has taken his research on sexual fantasies and explored why they are super normal and how to share them with a partner to make your sex life hotter.

Masturbation

Sex For One: The Joy of Selfloving by Betty Dodson, PhD (and all things Betty Dodson and Carlin Ross)

Betty is the OG badass, a fine artist whose interest in the women's liberation movement turned her into the guru of liberated sexuality. This book was first published as *Liberating Masturbation*, because she saw our culture of shame and silence as a form of repression. Reclaimed sexuality as political liberty? That idea totally has my vote!

In Your Hands: The Everyman's Guide to Masturbation by Mark Emme

Most resources out there are intended for cis women, but Mark Emme's book is full of techniques for cis men (and would apply to other individuals with penises), including practices for extended sessions and controlling ejaculation, and information on using the foreskin.

Getting Off: A Woman's Guide To Masturbation by Jamye Waxman

Includes great descriptions of every part of the vulva and vagina.

The Clitoral Truth: The Secret World at Your Fingertips by Rebecca Chalker

Fantastic information about more than just masturbation.

Orientation Spectrum

How to Understand Your Gender by Meg-John Barker and Alex Iantaffi

A comprehensive and compassionate guide to all the ways we might identify and express ourselves around gender.

Bi: Notes for a Bisexual Revolution by Shiri Eisner

A wonderful political treatise on the expanse of human sexuality. Really about all the ways we can be non-monosexual, not just bi.

You and Your Gender Identity: A Guide to Discovery by Dara Hoffman-Fox and Zinnia Jones

Dara is a clinician as well as being genderqueer, and this book is about exploration more than information. Parents of gender-questioning kiddos find this very helpful.

Asexuality: A Brief Introduction by Asexuality Archive

This is my go-to reference because it focuses on the voices and lived experience of ace individuals.

Stone Butch Blues by Les Feinberg

A classic novel bringing voice to and affirming the stone experience. Newly back in print and available for free public download.

Partnering Better

Hold Me Tight: Seven Conversations for a Lifetime of Love by Sue Johnson

A helpful book full of great ideas, though with some irritating self-help lingo, based in attachment theory.

How to Fight by Thich Nhat Hanh

This little book has great information about how mindfulness and kindness to ourselves allow us to let go of anger

10 Lessons To Transform Your Marriage: America's Love Lab Experts Share Their Strategies for Strengthening Your Relationship by John and Julie Gottman

The Gottmans have done decades of research on relationship configurations (I mentioned their four horsemen in this book) and have developed excellent strategies for communicating more effectively with your partner.

Polyamory

The Ethical Slut, Third Edition: A Practical Guide to Polyamory, Open Relationships, and Other Freedoms in Sex and Love by Janet W. Hardy and Dossie Easton

This is the classic book of the consensual non-monogamy movement and is still the one I recommend most. It has great information about negotiating all types of polyamory. While pro-polyam, the authors do talk about exploring hot monogamy as an option when one partner is deeply uncomfortable with polyamory.

Opening Up: A Guide to Creating and Sustaining Open Relationships by Tristan Taormino

Another great look at all the different ways polyamory can be used to increase relationship satisfaction.

Pornography and Sex "Addiction"

The Myth of Sex Addiction by David J. Ley

Unpacks all the research that shows why comparing sex and porn usage to other addictions is a false equivalence.

Ethical Porn for Dicks: A Man's Guide to Responsible Viewing Pleasure by David J. Ley

A Q&A format book created to help men find ways of viewing and using porn responsibly.

The Feminist Porn Book: The Politics of Producing Pleasure by Tristan Taormino

Features essays by feminists in the porn and sex industry along with feminist porn scholars, including a lot of positive uses of porn.

Self-Compassion

Self-Compassion: The Proven Power of Being Kind to Yourself by Kristin Neff

This book was enormously eye opening for me.

The Mindful Path to Self-Compassion: Freeing Yourself from Destructive Thoughts and Emotions by Christopher K. Germer

My other favorite book on self-compassion! Neff and Germer do a bunch of work together, too.

Sensate Focus

Sensate Focus in Sex Therapy: The Illustrated Manual by Linda Weiner and Constance Avery-Clark

A manual created for professionals on walking clients through sensate focus activities, but also a great resource if you are doing the work on your own.

The Complete Idiot's Guide to Sensual Massage by Patti Britton and Helen Hodgson

Patti Britton is a well known certified sex coach and sex educator who uses many of the principles of sensate focus in this self-help sensual massage book.

Sex and Gender Confirmation

Sex Without Roles: Transcending Gender by Eli Sachse

A zine about exploring your sexuality in a healthy way as you transition.

Trans Bodies, Trans Selves by Laura Erickson-Schroth

This comprehensive book has a whole chapter on intimate relationships.

The Trans Partner Handbook: A Guide For When Your Partner Transitions by Jo Green

Covers a ton of different topics related to partner transition, including possible changes to sex and sexuality.

Sex Toys/Sex Aids

The Big Book of Sex Toys: From Vibrators and Dildos to Swings and Slings--Playful and Kinky Bedside Accessories That Make Your Sex Life Amazing by Tristan Taormino

Tons of information for solo and partnered use plus photos to take the guesswork of how to actually make everything work!

The Many Joys of Sex Toys: The Ultimate How-to Handbook for Couples and Singles by Anne Semans

Another illustrated guide that covers toys and toy usage techniques. Think of it as a sex cookbook with the toys as the ingredients!

Oh Joy, Sex Toy by Erica Moen and Matthew Nolan

A webcomic and four (so far!) book volumes that cover all kinds of ways of having sex, solo and partnered, for all kinds of different bodies.

Sex While Parenting

Hump: True Tales of Sex After Kids by Kimberly Ford

A collection of honest essays about reclaiming sex after having children, including stories from a wide variety of couples.

The Mother's Guide to Sex: Enjoying Your Sexuality Through All Stages of Motherhood by Anne Semans and Cathy Winks

Lots of anecdotes and tips to draw from…whether your kids are 18 months or 18 years old!

Sex-Positive Parenting

Not Your Mother's Meatloaf: A Sex Education Comic Book by Saiya Miller and Liza Bley

Comics for youth that take away the shame and secretiveness of sex education without being dry and boring. This was the book I left sitting out for my own kids!

Woke Parenting by Bonnie Scott and Faith Harper

This zine did so well that it will soon become a book. All of us next-generation parents are desperate for materials that speak to our values and the modern world. How our children express themselves, their identities, and their bodies is a huge part of that.

Sexual Abuse

Things That Help by Cindy Crabb

Cindy's second zine compilation is some of my favorite writing about healing after sexual trauma, written by an incredibly articulate survivor. More at www.dorisdorisdoris. com.

Dear Sister: Letters From Survivors of Sexual Violence by Lisa Factora-Borchers

The letters are affirming and honest without veering off into being tragedy porn.

The Sexual Healing Journey: A Guide For The Survivors of Sexual Abuse by Wendy Maltz

A step by step guide on managing your trauma responses during sexual intimacy in order to reclaim a healthy, fulfilling sex life.

Spirituality

Sex, God, and the Conservative Church: Erasing Shame from Sexual Intimacy by Tina Schermer Sellers

A dense book meant for clinicians. But it has a brilliant history of Western culture and the lens of conservative religion and how that has impacted human sexuality with ideas on how to heal from the negative messages without giving up your faith tradition.

UnClobber: Rethinking Our Misuse of the Bible on Homosexuality by Colby Martin

My absolute favorite book ever on unpacking the "clobber" passages from the bible that are used to proclaim homosexuality as a sin. By an evangelical preacher whose story of coming to allyship is as important as his scriptural interpretation.

Trauma

Unfuck Your Brain by Faith Harper

I've distilled a lot of information about the physiological underpinnings of trauma and showed you how to work with it.

Waking The Tiger by Peter Levine

A great book on how the body holds trauma and how that impacts all domains of our lives.

References

"5 Reasons People Choose to Stay Single." *Psychology Today,* Sussex Publishers, www.psychologytoday.com/us/blog/me-we/201309/5-reasons-people-choose-stay-single.

Addington, D. (1997). *A hand in the bush.* San Francisco, CA: Greenery Press.

Addington, D. (2006). *Play piercing.* San Francisco, Calif.: Greenery.

Alman, I. (1993). *Let's talk sex.* Freedom, CA: Crossing Press.

Apps, A. (n.d.). *Intersex.*

arXiv, Emerging Technology from the. "The Way Strangers Meet via Dating Websites Is Changing Society in Unexpected Ways, Say Researchers." *MIT Technology Review, MIT Technology Review,* 10 Oct. 2017, www. technologyreview.com/s/609091/first-evidence-that-online-dating-is-changing-the-nature-of-society/.

Asexuality Archive. (2012). *Asexuality: A brief introduction.*

Barker, M. and Hancock, J. (n.d.). *Enjoy sex.*

Barker, M. and Scheele, J. (2016). *Queer.* London: Icon Books Ltd.

Barnes-Svarney, P. (2012). *Why Do Women Crave More Sex in the Summer?.* Penguin Group (USA) Incorporated.

Bass, E. and Davis, L. (1992). *The courage to heal.* New York: HarperPerennial.

Becker, G. (1997). *The gift of fear.* Boston: Little, Brown and Company.

Belge, K. and Bieschke, M. (2012). *Queer.* San Francisco, Calif.: Zest.

Berkowitz, E. (2013). *Sex and punishment*. Berkeley, Calif.: Counterpoint.

Bernstein, R. (2009). *The East, the West, and sex*. New York: Vintage Books.

Binaohan, B. (2014). *Decolonizing Trans/Gender 101*. biyuti publishing.

Blank, H. (2000). *Big big love*. Emeryville, CA: Greenery Press.

Blank, J. and Corinne, T. (2011). *Femalia*. San Francisco, CA: Last Gasp.

Blank, J. and Whidden, A. (2000). *Good vibrations*. San Francisco, Calif.: Down There Press.

Blue, V. (2006). *The adventurous couple's guide to sex toys*. San Francisco, Calif.: Cleis Press.

Blum, D. (2014). *Sex on the brain*. New York: Penguin Books.

Blume, E. (1998). *Secret survivors*. New York: Ballantine Books.

Bongiovanni, A., Jimerson, T., Crank! and Yarwood, A. (n.d.). *A quick & easy guide to they/them pronouns*.

Bornstein, K. (1220). *A queer and pleasant danger*. Boston, Mass: Beacon.

Bornstein, K. (2013). *Gender Outlaw*. Hoboken: Taylor and Francis.

Bornstein, K. and Bergman, S. (2010). *Gender outlaws*. Berkeley, CA: Seal Press.

Boyd, H. (2007). *She's not the man I married*. New York: Seal Press.

Breaking silence. (1995). New York: Xanthus Press.

Britton, P. and Lerma, H. (2003). *The complete idiot's guide to sensual massage illustrated*. Indianapolis, Ind.: Alpha.

Britton, P. (n.d.). *The art of sex coaching*.

Brody, M. (n.d.). *Stop the fight!*.

Campbell, D. "Body image concerns more men than women, research finds." *The Guardian* Jan. 6, 2012. https://www.theguardian.com/lifeandstyle/2012/jan/06/body-image-concerns-men-more-than-women

Carnes, P. (1989). *Contrary to love*. Minneapolis: CompCare.

Carnes, P. (1992). *Don't call it love*. New York: Bantam.

Carnes, P. (2001). *Facing the shadow*. Wickenburg, AZ: Gentle Path.

Carnes, P. and Carnes, P. (2001). *Out of the shadows*. Center City, MN: Hazelden Information & Edu.

Carnes, P. and Moriarity, J. (1997). *Sexual anorexia*. Center City (Minn.): Hazelden.

Carnes, P., Delmonico, D. and Griffin, E. (2008). *In the shadows of the net*. Center City, Minn.: Hazelden.

Castelman, Michael. "How much of porn depicts violence against women?" Psychology Today, June 15, 2016. https://www.psychologytoday.com/us/blog/all-about-sex/201606/how-much-porn-depicts-violence-against-women

Chodorow, N. (n.d.). *Femininities, masculinities, sexualities*.

Cockrill, K., Gimeno, L. and Herold, S. (2015). *Untold stories*. North Charleston: CreateSpace Independent Publishing Platform.

Cohen Greene, C. and Garano, L. (n.d.). *An intimate life*.

Corinna, H. (2007). *S.E.X*. New York: Da Capo.

Cottrell, S. (2014). *Mom, I'm gay*. [Place of publication not identified]: Freedhearts.

Davis, L. (1991). *Allies in healing*. New York, N.Y.: HarperPerennial.

Davis, L. (1991). *The courage to heal workbook*. New York, N.Y.: Harper & Row.

Diamond, L. (2009). *Sexual fluidity*. Cambridge, Mass.: Harvard University Press.

Diamond, M. (2011). *Trans/love*. San Francisco: Manic D Press.

Dodson, B. (1996). *Sex for one*. New York: Crown Trade Paperbacks.

Dohrenwend, A. (2012). *Coming around*. Far Hills, N.J.: New Horizon Press.

Dreisbach, S. "Shocking body image news" *Glamour*, Feb 2, 2011. https://www.glamour.com/story/shocking-body-image-news-97-percent-of-women-will-be-cruel-to-their-bodies-today

Duron, L. (2013). *Raising my rainbow*. New York: Broadway Books.

Durve, A. (2012). *The power to break free workbook*. [United States]: Power Press LLC.

Easton, D. and Hardy, J. (2004). *Radical ecstasy*. Oakland, Calif.: Greenery Press.

Easton, D. and Liszt, C. (n.d.). *The ethical slut*.

Easton, D., Hardy, J. and Easton, D. (2003). *The new topping book*. Oakland, CA: Greenery Press.

Easton, D., Liszt, C. and Beck, A. (1997). *The bottoming book, or, how to get terrible things done to you by wonderful people*. [Place of publication not identified]: Greenery.

Ehrensaft, D. (n.d.). *The gender creative child*.

Eisner, S. (n.d.). *Bi*.

Emberley, M. and Harris, R. (2009). *It's Perfectly Normal*. Somerville: Candlewick Press.

Emerson, D. (n.d.). *Trauma-sensitive yoga in therapy*.

Emme, M. (2013). *In your hands*. Berlin: Bruno Gmander.

Erickson-Schroth, L. (n.d.). *Trans bodies, trans selves*.

Evans, P. (2003). *Verbal abuse survivors speak out*. Holbrook, Mass.: Adams Media.

Factora-Borchers, L. and Simmons, A. (n.d.). *Dear sister*.

Feinberg, L. (2005). *Transgender warriors*. Boston, Mass: Beacon Press.

Feinberg, L. (2006). *Drag king dreams*. New York: Carroll & Graf Publishers.

Feinberg, L. (2007). *Trans liberation*. Boston, Mass: Beacon Press.

Fernbach, A. (2003). *Fantasies of fetishism*. New Brunswick, NJ [u.a.]: Rutgers Univ. Press.

Fields, R. Douglas (2015) *Why we snap*. New York: Dutton.

Fincham, F., Fernandes, L. and Humphreys, K. (1993). *Communicating in relationships*. Champaign, IL: Research Press.

Finley, K. (2000). *A different kind of intimacy*. New York: Thunder's Mouth Press.

Ford, J. (1997). *Child of the universe*. [Ellsworth, Me.]: [Epigrammata Press].

Forssberg, M. and Lundin, M. (2007). *Sex for guys*. Toronto [Ont.]: Groundwood Books.

Garbacik, J. and Lewis, J. (n.d.). *Gender & sexuality for beginners*.

Germer, C. (2009). *The mindful path to self-compassion*. New York: Guilford Press.

Glasser, W. (1995). *Staying together*. New York: HarperCollins.

Glenum, L. (2010). *Gurlesque*. Philadelphia, PA: Saturnalia Books.

Goad, J. (2007). *Jim Goad's gigantic book of sex*. Los Angeles, Calif.: Feral House.

Goldberg, S. and Brushwood Rose, C. (2009). *And Baby Makes More: Known Donors, Queer Parents, and Our Unexpected Families*. Insomniac Press.

Gottman, J., Gottman, J. and DeClaire, J. (n.d.). *Ten lessons to transform your marriage*.

Haberman, H. (n.d.). *Family jewels - a guide to male genital play and torment*.

Haines, S. (1999). *The survivor's guide to sex*. San Francisco: Cleis Press.

Hardy, J. (2006). *21st century kinkycrafts*. San Francisco, Calif.: Greenery.

Hasler, N. and Capozzola, M. (n.d.). *Sex*.

Heath, H. and White, I. (2002). *The challenge of sexuality in health care*. Osney Mead, Oxford: Blackwell Science.

Helminiak, D. (n.d.). *What the Bible really says about homosexuality*.

Henderson, E. and Armstrong, N. (n.d.). *100 questions you'd never ask your parents*.

Herek, G. (1998). *Stigma and sexual orientation*. London: SAGE.

Hills, R. (n.d.). *The sex myth*.

Hitt, S. (1997). *Cooking with less salt, less sugar, less fat ... in less time*. [Place of publication not identified]: Windmore Writers.

Hoffman-Fox, D., Jones, Z., Finch, S. and Keig, Z. (n.d.). *You and your gender identity*.

Hogan, S. (2003). *Gender issues in art therapy*. London: Jessica Kingsley Pub.

Holly, K. (n.d.). *Domestic violence safety plan*.

Hochschild, Arlie Russell. *The Managed Heart: Commercialization of Human Feeling*. University of California Press, 2012.

Jarvis, C. (2002). *The marriage sabbatical: the journey that brings you home*. Broadway Books/Jan.

Joannides, P., Gross, D. and Johnson, T. (n.d.). *Guide to getting it on*.

Johnson, S. (n.d.). *Hold me tight*.

Judson, O. (2003). *Dr. Tatiana's sex advice to all creation*. Metropolitan Owl Book.

Kahr, B. and Kahr, B. (2009). *Who's been sleeping in your head*. New York: Basic Books.

Karahassan, Philip. "How Technology Is Changing Dating." *PsychAlive*, 13 Sept. 2017, www.psychalive.org/how-technology-is-changing-dating/.